FUNDAMENTALS OF HEARING

FUNDAMENTALS OF HEARING
AN INSTRUCTOR'S WORKBOOK

William A. Yost

Parmly Hearing Institute
Loyola University Chicago
Chicago, Illinois

Academic Press
San Diego New York Boston
London Sydney Tokyo Toronto

Academic Press
A Harcourt Science and Technology Company
525 B Street, Suite 1900, San Diego, California 92101-4495, USA
http://www.academicpress.com

Academic Press Limited
Harcourt Place, 32 Jamestown Road, London NW1 7BY, UK
http://www.academicpress.com

Library of Congress Catalog Card Number: 00-103469

International Standard Book Number: 0-12-775696-5

PRINTED IN UNITED STATES OF AMERICA
00 01 02 03 04 05 SB 9 8 7 6 5 4 3 2 1

Fundamentals of Hearing: An Instructor's Workbook

Fundamentals of Hearing: An Instructor's Workbook

ABOUT THE WORKBOOK: This instructors workbook, the accompanying CD-ROM, and the web site at: *www.parmly.luc.edu* all compliment the book <u>Fundamentals of Hearing: An Introduction</u> (Fourth Edition, Academic Press, 2000). In order to derive the maximum benefit from the workbook and related materials, one should read and study <u>Fundamentals of Hearing: An Introduction</u>. The sixteen chapters in the workbook and at the web site, as well as the material on the CD-ROM are organized in the same manner as the sixteen chapters in the textbook. The Workbook and CD-ROM are intended for teachers using <u>Fundamentals of Hearing: An Introduction</u>.

<u>WORKBOOK</u>: This workbook contains two sections for each of the sixteen chapters:

1) An introduction containing a reminder about the CD-ROM and web site and suggested selections from the <u>Audio Demonstrations CD</u> produced by the Acoustical Society of America. The Introduction also contains *Instructional Hints* for each chapter.

2) A set of problems/questions and answers. Several workbook chapters contain general purpose figures to be used for testing student's knowledge on the chapter's subject matter.

The <u>Audio Demonstrations CD</u> is a selection of audio demonstrations on a compact disk (CD) produced by the Acoustical Society of America (ASA) and can be obtained by contacting the ASA at Suite 1N01, 2 Huntington Quadrangle, Melville, NY 11747-4502; (516) 576-2360, Fax: (516) 576-2377, e-mail: asa@aip.org.

<u>CD-ROM</u>: The CD-ROM contains the following files and programs:

1) A copy of all figures from <u>Fundamentals of Hearing: An Introduction</u>. Line drawings are in *. *gif* (CompuServe Bitmap) format and all photographs in *.*jpg* (JPEG Bitmap) format (These are found in the CD-ROM directory: *Figures,* and are listed by chapter. Read the **readFig.txt** file for more information).

2) All data in all data figures and the data for all waveform and spectral figures used in <u>Fundamentals of Hearing: An Introduction</u> are provided in delimited ASCII text (*.*txt*) format that can be read into almost all wordprocessors and spread sheets (These are found in the CD-ROM directory: *DataTxt,* and are listed by chapter. Read the **readTxt.txt** file for more information).

3) The Figures from each chapter of <u>Fundamentals of Hearing: An Introduction</u> are provided as Microsoft PowerPoint presentation (*.*pps*) files (These are found in the CD-ROM directory:

PwrPtFigs, and are listed by chapter. Read the **readPpt.txt** file for more information).

4) A "toolbox" of MATLAB functions for generating, playing, and analyzing sounds (These are found in the directory: *MATTools*. Read the **readMat.txt** file for more information).

5) Three executable programs that can be run in Windows 95, Windows 98, and NT. One program (**Sound Generator**) is for generating, listening to, and graphing simple and complex sound waveforms, one program (**Neural**) is a simulation of obtaining an input-output function from an auditory nerve fiber and allows one to generate tuning curves and neural response areas, and one program (**2AFC**) is a general purpose program that allows one to perform two-alternative, forced-choice listening experiments based on stimuli generated with **Sound Generator**. (These are found in the directory: *Programs* and its three subdirectories. Read the **readPrg.txt** file in Programs for more information.)

The CD-ROM is for PC based computers running Windows 95, 98, or NT and it is designed for computers with sound cards. Access to wordprocessing, spread sheets, Microsoft PowerPoint, MATLAB, and graphic programs that can read **.gif* and **.jpg* figure files are also necessary to take full advantage of the CD-ROM., although each section of the CD-ROM contains useful material. More details for each of the five sets of files and programs can be found in the *"readXXX.txt"* (readFig, readTxt, readPpt, readMat, readPrg) files located in each directory of the CD-ROM. These are ASCII text (**.txt*) files that can be read by any wordprocessor. The CD-ROM is to be used to download the desired files and programs for use by the instructor.

To access to CD-ROM, place the CD in the CD reader. Then, either copy the files to a folder on your computer's hard drive for your use, or access the files from the CD as if the CD were another disk drive, or use the setup.exe programs as described in the readPrg.txt file in the directory *Programs*. Additional details contained in some of the readXXX.txt files found in each directory.

WEB SITE: The web site at *www.parmly.luc.edu* is located at the Parmly Hearing Institute of Loyola University Chicago. The **Hearing Tutorial** web site contains information about Fundamentals of Hearing: An Introduction and Fundamentals of Hearing: An Instructor's Workbook. The main section of the web site contains sixteen chapters with interactive demonstrations highlighting many, *but not all*, of the points made in the textbook Fundamentals of Hearing: An Introduction. While the demonstrations are primarily designed for use with Fundamentals of Hearing: An Introduction, many of them can be used without reference to this textbook. The web site also contains links to other educational and related material dealing with hearing and the related senses.

Windows 95, Windows 98, NT and PowerPoint are products of Microsoft Corporation. MATLAB is a product of Math Works, Inc.

Chapter 1 - The World We Hear

CD-ROM, Web Site, ASA Tapes: The CD-ROM and Web Site (*www.parmly.luc.edu/*) should be consulted.

Instructional Hints: Al Bregman's concept of an auditory scene is a useful way of describing a complex acoustic environment (*Auditory Scene Analysis*, MIT Press, 1991). Just like a visual scene is the perception of visual objects, so is an auditory scene the perception of sound sources.

It is probably worth mentioning the Appendix to the book as a place for the student to go if they feel they do not have sufficient background on a topic.

This chapter mixes physical attributes such as frequency with subjective ones such as pitch. The differences are mentioned in Chapter 2.

Using the proper experimental design and control is something a scientist learns over time. An example that captures many students' attention deals with the "vacuum-cleaner salesman's pitch." While the example is not an experiment per se, it makes several points about confounding variables and experimental control:

After you have just bought a very good vacuum cleaner and before you have even had a chance to use it, your doorbell rings. A salesman throws dirt on your rug, and asks you to clean it up with your vacuum cleaner. He says to take as long as you like. He then uses his new cleaner. He shows you that his vacuum cleaner has picked up a lot of the dirt that, presumably, your cleaner missed. There are no tricks with the demonstration. Is his vacuum cleaner better? Not necessarily!

The "experiment" needs to be done in the other order. He cleans up the dirt first, then you follow, and then vice versa. One then compares the amount of dirt in the two vacuum cleaners. The confound is a "time-reversal confound." This example makes several points: 1) Determining confounding variables can be subtle, 2) Finding confounding variables often requires that the experimenter know a lot about the topic under study. In this case, the time-reversal confound is something to control for since it is almost impossible to remove all of the dirt from a rug, unless it is placed in a complete vacuum, 3) Determining the proper control for a confounding variable is often obvious once the confounding variable is identified.

Chapter 1 - Suggested Problems for Students

1) What three attributes of sound are coded by the *auditory periphery*?

2) What are the differences between the studies of *anatomy* and *physiology*?

3) At what stage of "hearing" is sound source determination most likely to occur and why?

4) Which type of clinician would most likely attend to the following hearing problems?

     A) An ear infection

     B) Courses in lip reading

     C) Hearing aid fitting

5) What are the two classical theories of "hearing"?

6) In the following description of a <u>hypothetical</u> experiment determine the *I.V.*, the *D.V.*, the *C.V.*, and write out an equation for the *functional relationship* between the *D.V.* and the *I.V.* Explain how the *C.V.* was controlled for.

     This experiment concerns the effect of age on hearing loss. The amount of hearing loss was measured in 6 groups of people: 10 people between 10 and 20 years old, 10 between 20 and 30 years, 10 between 30 and 40 years, 10 between 40 and 50 years, 10 between 60 and 70 years, and 10 between 70 and 80 years. Because it had been shown that hearing loss differs between males and females, an equal number of males and females were assigned to each group. The study showed that average hearing loss in units of percent hearing loss [P(HL)] could be approximately predicted by multiplying one's age (A) by 1.4 and then subtracting 9% from this product (the prediction was only accurate for ages up to 72 years).

7) From the *functional relationship* described in problem 6), provide a *Table* and a *Figure* of the results when the I.V. takes on values from 20 to 60 in steps of 10.

Answers for Problems for CHAPTER 1

1) *Frequency, intensity, and time* are the physical attributes of sound.

2) *Anatomy* is the study of the structure of the parts of the body, while *physiology* is the study of the biological function of these parts.

3) Sound source determination would most likely occur beyond the coding stage since the information needed to determine sound sources must come from the neural code.

4) An *otologist (otolaryngologist, ENT doctor)* would treat middle ear infections, an *audiologist* would provide lip reading training, and either an otologist or audiologist could fit a hearing aid (this is most often done by an audiologist).

5) The *place theory* of von Bekesy and the *temporal or volley theory* of Wever.

6) *D.V.* = hearing loss or P(HL), *I.V.* = age of person according to the six age groups, *C.V.* = gender, P(HL) = 1.4(A$_{in\ years}$) - 9%, and the effect of gender was controlled for by having the same number of males and females in each of the six groups.

7) Table. The mean percent hearing loss [P(HL)] for different ages (in years).

Age	P(HL)
20 years	19%
30	33%
40	47%
50	61%
60	75%

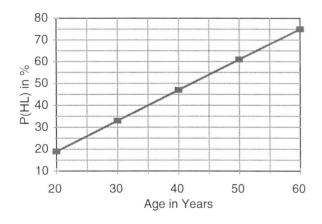

Figure. Percent hearing loss [P(HL)] as a function of age in years

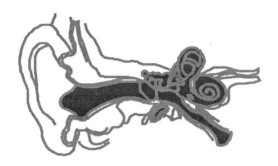

Chapter 2 - Sinusoids, The Basic Sound

CD-ROM, Web Site, ASA Tapes: The CD-ROM and Web Site (*www.parmly.luc.edu/*) should be consulted.

<u>ASA Tapes:</u> Demonstration 6, Track 17, 18; Demonstration 12, Track 27, 28. Although these demonstrations cover topics relevant to the psychophysics of pitch and loudness, they can be used to demonstrate frequency and amplitude for pure tones.

Instructional Hints: Appendix A in the Textbook can be used to help students understand the relationship between the sinwave functions that are drawn in the Textbook and the trigonometric sin function. Start with the unit circle and the definition of the sin of the angle (i.e., the side opposite the angle divided by the hypotenuse). If the angle is zero, the side opposite has zero height, and, thus, the sin of the angle is zero (i.e., starting phase is zero). When the angle is 90°, the side opposite equals the hypotenuse, and, thus, the sin of 90° is 1. As you continue around the circle, the sin of each angle will form the zero-degree starting phase sinusoid, such as shown in Figure 2.1 in the Textbook.

It is sometimes useful to start with the older definition of frequency, which is cycles per second (cps), and then point out that in the 1950s the term cps was replaced by hertz to honor a famous German physicist, Heinrich Hertz (1857-1894), who studied electromagnetism.

It is crucial to communicate to the student that starting phase is a relative value, and that the zero-degree starting condition is a convention. It might also be worthwhile pointing out that a circle can also be divided into radians, and there are 2π radians in a circle (i.e., thus π radians equals 180°).

It is often said that the auditory system is phase insensitive (a statement sometimes attributed to Helmholtz). This is true for a long-duration sinwave. That is, there are no perceptual changes when the starting phase of a long-duration sinwave is changed. However, there are many situations (e.g., interaural phase differences, or comparing a harmonic series added with the same versus random phases, etc.) in which changes in starting phases are very perceptible. Thus, it is probably best to avoid the statement that the auditory system is phase insensitive.

For the students who do not know what an integral is, explaining that it is the area under a function helps explain why the integral of a sinwave is zero, but the integral of a sinwave squared (i.e., as in the definition of rms) is never zero. For those who know some statistics, rms is the standard deviation of a variable with zero mean (i.e., a sinwave has a zero mean, and it is symmetric about zero displacement). Sounding out the term "rms" helps describe the operations, i.e, the "<u>r</u>oot" (square root) of the "<u>m</u>ean" of the "<u>s</u>quared" amplitudes.

The mass and spring example is often used as a model for air molecules, which will be introduced in Chapter 2 of the Textbook. The solution of the mass and spring relationship is the common wave equation for describing sound in a medium.

There is a conceptual gap that students sometimes have trouble with. If something vibrates slowly (e.g., at 1 Hz), then the perception is of something changing once per second. As the frequency increases, the rate of change increases until at some rate (around 20 Hz) there is no longer a perception of change, but a stable unchanging "sound." If the vibration pattern is simple and is repeated periodically, the sound takes on a pitch, and the pitch then increases as the rate of vibration increases beyond 20 Hz. The difference between the perception of something changing to a stabilized sound percept with a pitch is the frequency range where hearing begins. Understanding the mechanism of stabilization is an interesting challenge for theories of auditory perception (see Patterson et al. 1995).

Patterson, R. D., Allerhand, M., & Giguere, C. (1995). Time domain modeling of peripheral auditory processing: A modular architecture and a software platform. *Journal of the Acoustical Society of America, 98*, 1890-1894.

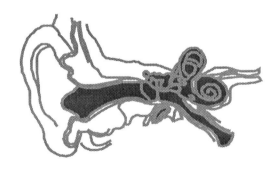

Chapter 2 - Suggested Problems for Students

1) *INSTRUCTOR: The figures at the end of this section can be used to quiz students about amplitude, frequency, and starting phase.*

2) Why can't sound travel in a vacuum?

3) What is missing in the following equation of a sin wave?

$$F(t) = B \sin(2\pi t)$$

4) Can you draw a sinusoid with a peak amplitude of 5 and a period of 1 ms? If not, why not?

5) Correct the following sentences:

a) Mr. Jones perceived the frequency of the violin in the orchestra.

b) The frequency meter indicated that the car produced a high pitch.

c) The noise meter indicated that the airplane was loud.

d) The wind sounded as if it varied in amplitude as it became night.

6) Plot this waveform and determines its peak, peak-to-peak, and rms amplitude; and its period and repetition frequency:

Time:	0.1ms	0.2ms	0.3ms	0.4ms	0.5ms	0.6ms	0.7ms	0.8ms	0.9ms	1.0ms
Instantaneous Amplitude (cm):	0	3	-2	-5	-1	0	3	-2	-5	-1

7) Draw two complete cycles of a sin wave that has a frequency of 100 Hz, peak amplitude of 1 cm, and a starting phase of $0°$.

8) On the same axis as used for question 7) draw a sin wave with the same peak amplitude and starting phase as that used in problem 7) but with twice the frequency (draw four cycles of this higher-frequency sinusoid). What is the instantaneous phase difference between the two sinusoids at 5 ms and at 20 ms?

9) What would happen to the two phase differences at 5 and 10 ms in problem 8) if the higher frequency sinusoid had a 180° starting phase rather than a 0° starting phase?

10) A sin wave has a peak-to-peak amplitude of 16 cm, what is its peak and rms amplitude?

11) Draw two cycles of a cosine wave with a frequency of 500 Hz and an rms amplitude of 14.14 cm.

12) Draw four cycles of a damped sinusoid of 100 Hz, peak amplitude of 9 cm, and starting phase of 90°. The damping changes by a factor of 1/3.

13) The two waveforms (A and B) shown below describe the vibration of two different objects. Which one encountered the greater friction? Why?

14) Describe the differences you might expect if the same mass and spring as shown in Fig. 2.10 of the Textbook were put in motion by the same force but the spring in case A was stiffer than that used for case B.

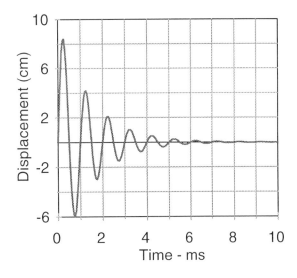

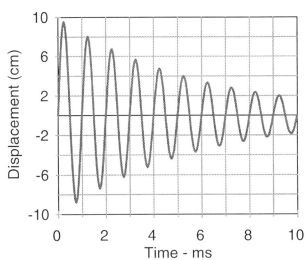

A   B

ADVANCED PROBLEMS

1) One oscillating object had three times the mass and half the stiffness of a second oscillating object. By what factor did the object's frequency change?

2) If w equals 628.31853 radians/sec, what is the frequency of oscillation?

3) What is the rms amplitude of a cosinusoid wave with peak amplitude, A?

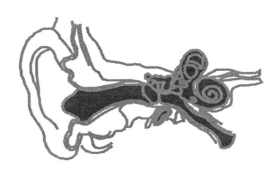

Answers for Problems for CHAPTER 2

1) *On the first page in the upper left is 4 cylces of a 200-Hz, 10-cm peak, 0° sinwave; upper right is 8 cycles of a 400-Hz, 4-cm peak, 180° sinwave; lower left is 2 cycles of a 50-Hz, 100-cm peak, 90° sinwave, and lower right is 3 1/4 cycles of a 500-Hz, 2-cm peak, 45° sinwave. On the second page are the same sinwaves without axis numbers (b from page 1 is a, a from page 1 is b, d from page 1 is c, and c from page 1 is d)*

2) Since a vacuum means the absence of any particles, there are no objects with mass to vibrate.

3) Both the frequency, f, and the starting phase, θ, are missing.

4) No, the sinusoid cannot be drawn since starting phase is not specified.

5) Correct sentences are:

a) Mr. Jones perceived the <u>pitch</u> (not frequency) of the violin in the orchestra.

b) The frequency meter indicated that the car produced a high <u>frequency</u> (not pitch).

c) The noise meter indicated that the airplane <u>had a high amplitude</u> (not was loud).

d) The wind sounded as if varied in <u>loudness</u> (not amplitude) as it became night.

6) The peak amplitude is 3 cm, peak-to-peak is 8 cm, and
$rms = 0^2+3^2+-2^2+-5^2+-1^2 = 9+4+25+1 = 39; 39/5 = 7.8; \sqrt{7.8} = 2.79$ cm.

Period = 0.5 ms, frequency =1000/.5=2000 Hz.

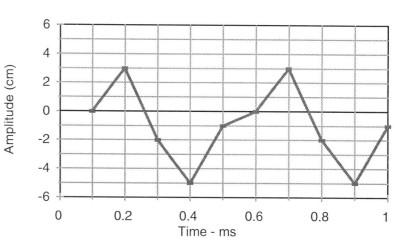

7)

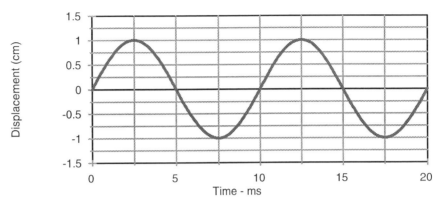

8) At 5 ms the instantaneous phase difference is 180° and at 20 ms it is 0°.

9) Phases reverse, so that at 5 ms the difference is 0° and at 20 ms it is 180°.

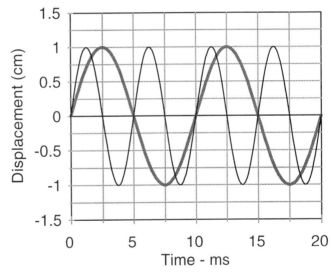

10) Peak amplitude is 8 cm and rms is 5.656 (8x0.707).

11) Cosine means 90° starting phase, and an rms amplitude of 14.14 cm yields a peak amplitude of 20 cm (i.e., if $A_{rms}=.707A$, then $A=A_{rms}/.707$).

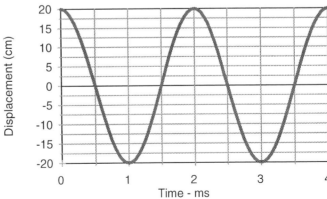

12)

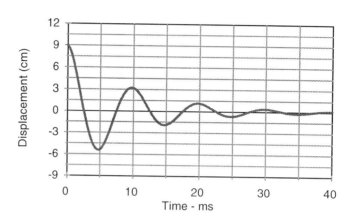

13) "A" has the greater friction since the waveform damps more quickly.

14) A stiffer spring would reduce the amplitude and increase the frequency.

ADVANCED PROBLEMS

1) $f = \sqrt{(s/m)}$, $\sqrt{(0.5s/3m)} = \sqrt{[(0.5/3)(s/m)]} = \sqrt{(0.1666(s/m))} = 0.40824(\sqrt{s/m})$

2) $f = 100$ Hz

3) Since $\sin 90° - wt = \cos wt$, then the same calculations as were used in the Supplement Section may be used by substituting $(90° - wt)$ for (wt), and since adding $90°$ of phase does not change the evaluation of the integrals, the rms amplitude is still $A/\sqrt{2}$.

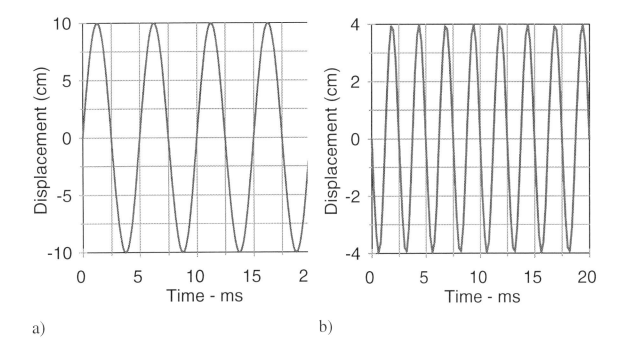

a)   b)

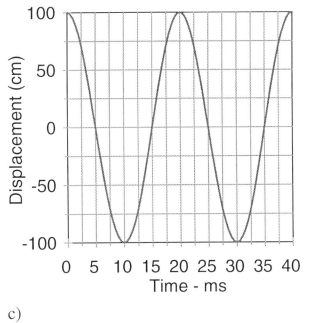

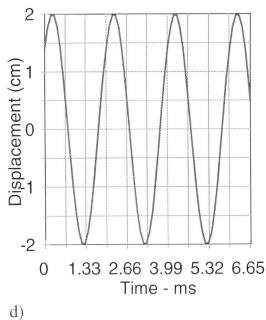

c)   d)

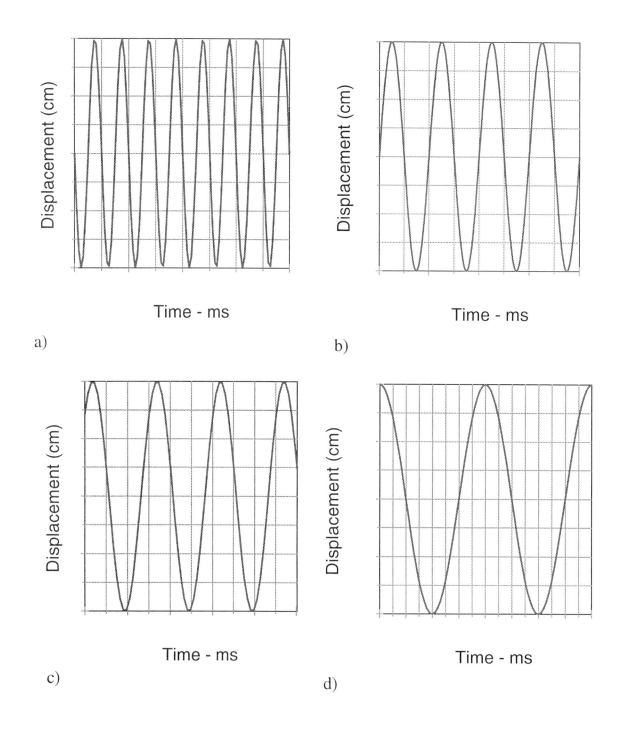

a)

Time - ms

b)

Time - ms

c)

Time - ms

d)

Time - ms

Chapter 3 - Sound Transmission

CD-ROM, Web Site, ASA Tapes: The CD-ROM and Web Site (*www.parmly.luc.edu/*) should be consulted.
ASA Tapes: Demonstration 4, Track 8,11. Although these demonstrations cover topics relevant to the psychophysics of loudness, they can be used to demonstrate the decibel.

Instructional Hints: While one has to be cautious about the analogy of using water to describe wave motion in air, a pan of water is a useful way to make many points about wave propagation, rarefactions, condensations, and wavelength. A piece of rope about 6 feet long is also useful for standing wave demonstrations.

The Table shown below might be useful in making decibels relevant.

Sound Intensity (watts/cm^2)	Sound Pressure (µPa)	dB SPL	Possible Sound Source
10^{-2} (0.01)	200,000,000	140	Ear-drum damage
10^{-4} (0.0001)	20,000,000	120	Next to a jet engine
10^{-6}	2,000,000	100	Peak level at a ball game
10^{-8}	200,000	80	Very loud shout
10^{-10}	20,000	60	Normal conversation
10^{-12}	2,000	40	Very quiet room
10^{-14}	200	20	Sound-proof room
10^{-16}	20	0	Thresholds of hearing

Students should be reminded to check the units of measurement when they make calculations. In addition to providing a more meaningful understanding, such calculations can often help check an answer.

Using a simple musical recorder and changing its pitch by covering different note holes helps make the connection between length of tubes and standing waves.

Chapter 3 - Suggested Problems for Students

1) Sound depends on objects that have inertia and elasticity. When sound travels from its source to our ears, what are the objects that would vibrate?

2) Explain how a vibrating object sets up regions of *condensation* and *rarefaction* in the air.

3) What is the difference between the period and the wavelength of a sound wave?

4) If the speed of a 1,000-Hz sound is 400 meters per second, what is the sound's wavelength (make sure the units of wavelength are correct)?

5) In the old west, Native Americans would put their ears to the ground to detect the presence of a faraway herd of running buffalo. Why did they "listen" to the sound traveling through the ground rather than through the air?

6) What causes the pressure in a filled balloon to be higher than that of an empty balloon? In which balloon would sound travel faster? Why?

7) If at one moment in time a three gram object is traveling with a velocity of 6 cm per sec, what is the pressure this object would exert in a 9-cm^2 area (again, make sure the units of measurement are correct, check the units against those shown in Table 3.1 in the Textbook)?

8) The weight of a person exerts some force (F) on the ground. Which woman would produce more pressure on the ground at the heel of her shoe: a 100-lb women wearing flat-heel shoes or a100-lb women wearing spiked-heel shoes? Why?

9) If it takes 2400 joules of energy to cook an egg and the power of the burner on your stove is 20 joules/sec, how long will it take to cook the egg?

10) A loudspeaker is vibrating at 20 Hz and the amplitude of vibration is very high. I take a light piece of paper and hold it a foot or so in front of the loudspeaker. The paper vibrates in my hand. Why is it vibrating and at what frequency is it likely to be vibrating? (You might want to try this sort of "experiment" with your stereo system. Just make sure your neighbors are tolerant).

11) Convert the following ratios into decibels of energy:

   a) 1, b) 0.1, c) 2, d) 0.001, e) 400, f) 1,600, g) 0.015, h) 150,000

16

12) Convert the following decibels into pressure ratios:

      a) 0 dB, b) 10 dB, c) -6 dB, d) 35 dB, e) -13 dB

13) A person with good hearing can detect a 500-Hz tone coming from a headphone that exerts 100 μPa of sound pressure. How much pressure (in units of μPa) could a person with a 20-dB hearing loss detect? If the threshold for hearing is 10 dB SPL for the person with good hearing, what is the threshold for hearing for the person with the hearing loss?

14) You buy a stereo that the dealer says can put out 100 dB. Your friend buys one that he says puts out 120 dB. It turns out that both stereos put out the same sound pressure level. How can that be? (Hint: in each case the level in decibels is stated without a referent.)

15) When air molecules collide with each other in their random movement (called Brownian motion) the collisions create sound. Suppose the intensity of this sound is 30 dB below the softest sound humans can hear. If the softest sound humans can hear is approximately 10^{-16} watts/cm^2, what is the sound intensity of Brownian motion?

16a) Hypothetically, assume that the normal thresholds for hearing are 0 dB SPL for all frequencies. What are the thresholds (dB SPL) for hearing at each frequency for the person who has the type of hearing loss described below (dB HL means decibels of hearing loss or the number of decibels <u>above</u> the normal thresholds for hearing):

250 Hz = -5 dB HL, 500 Hz = 15 dB HL, 1000 Hz = 20 dB HL, 2000 Hz = 30 dB HL, 4000 Hz = 50 dB HL.

16b) Hypothetically, assume that 20 dB SPL is the normal threshold for hearing for all frequencies. If the values given below are the sound pressure levels that a person can detect at each frequency, how much hearing loss (dB HL) does this person have at each frequency:

250 Hz = 10 dB SPL, 500 Hz = 5 dB SPL, 1000 Hz = 20 dB SPL, 2000 Hz = 30 dB SPL, 4000 Hz = 50 dB SPL.

17) I am about to build a house near a noisy street. The front of my lot is 100 feet from the street and the back is 500 feet away. How many decibels will I reduce the level of the noise if I build my house at the back of the lot instead of at the front of the lot?

18) I want to build my house so that it is as soundproof as possible. Should I buy material with a high or low characteristic impedance (Zc)? Why?

19) Suppose I increase the stiffness of the spring in the mass-spring example shown in Figure 2.10 in the Textbook and discussed in the Chapter 3 (i.e., I increase the spring reactance). Will this increase or decrease the impedance to the motion of the mass, and will this increase or decrease the sound intensity that the moving mass would be able to produce? Explain.

20) Fluid in the middle ear acts like resistance for the parts of the middle ear that must vibrate when sound enters the middle ear. If I am told that I have fluid in my middle ear, would it be harder for me to hear some frequencies and not others ? Explain. If some structure in the middle ear were like a mass and it was operating abnormally, would it make a difference as to how well I could hear different frequencies? Explain. If the mass reactance increased with increasing frequency, would I be able to hear low or high frequencies better? Explain.

21) There is a high-pitched sound that is coming from somewhere in your kitchen. As you move around the kitchen in an attempt to locate the source of this sound, the sound is sometimes loud and sometimes so soft you can barely hear it. What might be happening?

22) A sound source is placed near your left ear about 30 cm away. I measure the sound pressure at your left ear and also at your right ear and then three meters further away from your right ear. What should I expect the differences to be between the measurements made at the left ear and the two made at the right ear? Explain.

23) As an architectural designer you are asked to suggest what to do about the poor sound quality of a small auditorium. Your measurements show that the reverberation time in the auditorium is very long. You know that this would lead to poor sound quality. Why? What might you do to shorten the reverberation time if you cannot change the size of the auditorium?

24) The outer ear canal is approximately 2.5 cm long. As a tube-like structure a standing wave can be set up in the canal when sound is present. Assuming that the canal is open only at one end, what would the fundamental frequency of the mode of the standing wave be (assume the speed of sound is 32,500 cm/sec)?

ADVANCED PROBLEMS

1) Explain the differences between a high-frequency sound and a sound that travels through air at a high speed.

2) What must be done to the mass of an object if one wants to increase its frequency of vibration by a factor of 9?

3) Two sinwaves of the same frequency are added. One wave has 10 units of peak amplitude and a starting phase of 45°, and the other has 5 units of peak amplitude and a starting phase of 135°. What are the amplitude and starting phase of the summed sinwave?

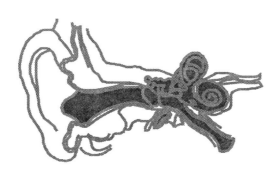

Answers for Problems for CHAPTER 3

1) The parts of the medium through which the sound travels. If this is air, then the molecules that make up air (e.g., oxygen, hydrogen, etc.) are the vibrating objects.

2) A condensation occurs when the air molecules are pushed in one direction at one time. A rarefaction occurs when the object pushing the molecules moves away from the molecules providing a vacant space which the molecules fill in obeying the principle of the gas laws so that the molecules fill the space evenly.

3) Period is the TIME it takes a waveform to complete one cycle. Wavelength is the DISTANCE between successive points on a wave traveling from a vibrating source. Since $f = 1/Pr$, and $\lambda = c/f$ ($f = c/\lambda$); then $c/\lambda = 1/Pr$; $\lambda = Pr/c$.

4) $\lambda = c/f$, $\lambda = (400 \text{ meters/sec})/(1000 \text{ cycles/sec}) = 0.4 \text{ meters} = 40 \text{ cm}$.

5) The sound from the distant herd will reach the listener sooner through the ground then through the air.

6) The density of the air molecules is greater in the filled balloon, and thus there is a greater mass exerting its force on the surface area of the balloon. Sound would travel faster through the filled balloon, since the density of the air molecules is greater.

7) $p = mv/tA$, $p = (3 \text{ grams})(6 \text{ cm/sec})/ 9 \text{ cm}^2 \text{ x sec} = 2 \text{ grams /cm x sec}^2$

8) The women wearing high heels, since the area at the bottom of the high heel is smaller than that of the flat heel. As the area gets smaller for the same force, the pressure gets higher.

9) $E = PT$, $T = E/P$, 2400 joules / 20 joules/sec = 120 sec or 2 minutes.

10) The paper is vibrating because the wave motion of the loudspeaker cone is being propagated through the air to the paper. Since the frequency of vibration is not affected by sound propagation, the paper would probably vibrate at 20 Hz.

11) Ratio | dB, energy [10log(ratio)]

Ratio	dB, energy [10log(ratio)]
1	0 dB
0.1	-10 dB
2	3.01 dB
0.001	-30 dB
400	26.02 dB
1600	32 dB
0.015	-18.24 dB
150,000	51.76 dB

12)

dB, pressure	Ratio [$10^{(dB/20)}$]
0 dB	1
10 dB	3.16
-6 dB	.501
35 dB	56.23
-13 dB	.224

13) 20 dB is a ratio of 10, 10(100 μPa) = 1000 μPA. 30 dB SPL is the threshold for the person with a 20 dB hearing loss.

14) The two measures of the decibel rating are referenced to different values. Since decibels is a ratio of one sound level referenced to another sound level, a sound can have a different decibel measure if it is compared to a different referent.

15) 30 dB is a ratio of 10^{-3} in intensity units; 10^{-3} X 10^{-16} = 10^{-19} watts/cm^2 is the sound intensity of Brownian motion.

16a)

HL	SPL
-5 dB	-5 dB
15 dB	15 dB
20 dB	20 dB
30 dB	30 dB
50 dB	50 dB

16b)

SPL	HL
10 dB	-10 dB
5 dB	-15 dB
20 dB	0 dB
30 dB	10 dB
50 dB	30 dB

17) The back is five times further, so r=5, r^2 =25, 10log25=13.97 dB is the reduction in level.

18) High characteristic impedance, since the higher the impedance difference between the material and air, the more the sound will be reflected off of the material.

19) If the spring reactance (Xs) increases, impedance decreases, from $Z=\sqrt{[R^2 +(Xm-Xs)^2)]}$.

20) Fluid would probably make it hard to hear all frequencies, since the impedance caused by resistance does not depend on frequency. Mass reactance is different for different frequencies, so an abnormality in mass would mean that the hearing problem would be different at different frequencies. If mass reactance increased with increasing frequency, then high frequencies would be harder to hear.

21) As one moves around in the kitchen, the sound at one location may be reinforced by a reflection and, thus, it might be loud at that point, whereas at a different location the reflective wave may act to partially cancel the originating sound, resulting in a softer sound at that location.

22) If the sound is measured close to one ear and close to the other ear, then the head may act as a sound shadow, and the sound at the ear opposite the source (right ear) may be low. As one moves the sound source away from this ear, the head will produce less of a shadow and the sound measured at this ear will increase and will eventually be nearly the same (except for the inverse square law) as that measured at the other ear (i.e., that near the source).

23) Increase the ability for the walls, floors, ceilings, etc. of the auditorium to absorb the sound, since reverberation time is inversely proportional to the amount of absorption.

24) fo=c/4L, fo = 32,500cm/sec / (4* 2.5 cm) = 32500/10 = 3,250 Hz.

ADVANCED PROBLEMS

1) At high frequencies sound oscillates or vibrates many times per second. For a fixed amplitude, the velocity of motion through one cycle at any one point in space is faster for a high-frequency sound than for a low-frequency sound. The speed of sound refers to the time it takes sound to propagated from one point in space to the next point independent of the sound's frequency.

2) Since frequency is related to the inverse of the square root of mass, a nine-fold increase in vibration means a three-fold decrease in mass.

3) Using vector addition and the law of cosines and noting that the phase difference is 90°; $R = \sqrt{(10^2 + 5^2 + 2x5x10xcos(90°))}$, cos(90°) = 0; $R=\sqrt{(100+25)}=\sqrt{125}=11.18$ units.

Chapter 4 - Complex Stimuli

CD-ROM, Web Site, ASA Tapes: The CD-ROM and Web Site (*www.parmly.luc.edu/*) should be consulted.
<u>ASA Tapes:</u> Demonstration 28, Track 53. Although these demonstrations cover topics relevant to timbre, they can be used to demonstrate harmonics and complex stimuli.

Instructional Hints: It is important to remind students that either the time domain or the frequency domain can be used to completely define a sound. One domain is not better than another. Which one is used depends on what type of information one wants to convey. Beats clearly show the importance of the time domain description for hearing. To make the point about the importance of the frequency domain, have the students imagine what they would hear if two very different notes of a piano are played at the same time (or play such notes). Students will hopefully realize that they hear two pitches. As such, the auditory system must have analyzed the complex waveform into two components corresponding to the two pitches. The ability to do this is similar to analyzing the complex waveform in the frequency domain.

If you have access to a sinwave generator, then a good demonstration is to play a low-frequency tone like a 100-Hz tone with a long duration, say 1 or 2 sec, without a rise/fall time to shape the onsets and offsets of the tone. Start the demonstration at a high level where the 100-Hz pitch is clearly perceived, then lower the level. At a fairly low level, the 100-Hz pitch will no longer be perceived, but a click sound will occur at the onset and offset of the tone. The perception of the clicks, but not the tone, is because the auditory system is not as sensitive to 100 Hz as it is to higher frequencies where the energy is spread to due to the sudden onsets and offsets of the tone.

One way to make the point that the spectrum of a pulsed tone is not a simple line at the frequency of the tone is to point out that the time domain description that one wants to obtain is one that contains no amplitude, then the sinwave, then no amplitude. A single-tone spectrum is a tone that is on forever.

If you want to show the long-term spectrum of an FM sinusoid, then consider an FM tone where $\beta = (m/F_m) = 1$. The figure below shows the amplitude spectrum. However, the spectra change, sometimes considerably, when the parameters of the FM tone are changed, making it impossible to state simple rules for determining FM spectra.

Some time should be spent explaining the log frequency axis of Figure 4.14 in the Textbook, since this sometimes confuses students and many log axes will be used in later chapters.

When covering spectrographs, you might want the students to look at Figure 14.10 in the Textbook to see an example of a speech spectrograph.

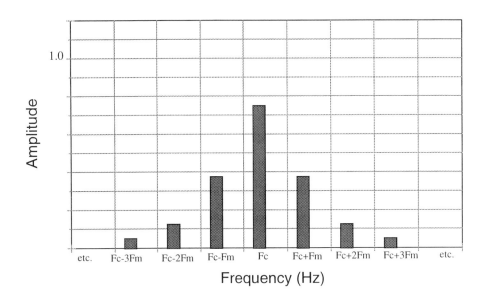

As problem 16 suggests, the average rate of envelope fluctuations for a narrow band noise is 2/3 times the bandwidth of the noise. As pointed out in the Supplement to the Textbook, the greater the level of a Gaussian noise, the greater the standard deviation of the normal distribution, which in terms of Figure 4.16 in the Textbook means that the peak level of the instantaneous amplitude of the noise will increase as level increases.

Chapter 4 - Suggested Problems for Students

1) Draw the time (two cycles) and frequency domain descriptions of a 500-Hz sinusoid with a peak amplitude of 100 v and a starting phase of 270°.

2) Suppose a 1,000-Hz sinusoid with a peak amplitude of 100 v and a starting phase of 0° is added to the waveform described in problem 1. Again draw the time and frequency domain descriptions of this complex waveform consisting of the sum of the two sinwaves (use two cycles of the 500-Hz tone and sixteen equally spaced points on the time domain waveforms).

3) Draw the time domain (3 cycles) waveform for the frequency domain description shown below.

Amplitude Spectrum

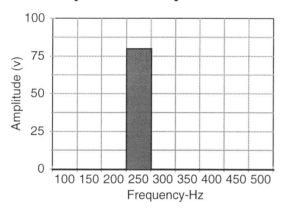

Phase Spectrum

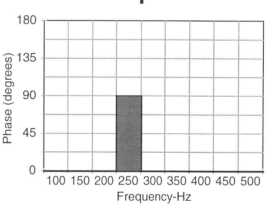

4) Using the time domain waveform that you derived in problem 2 as a guide, what are the frequencies of the two sinusoids that were added together to produce the complex waveform shown at the right.

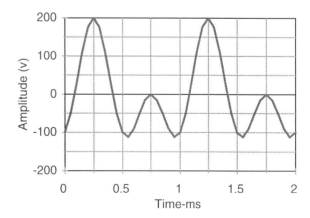

5) Draw the amplitude spectrum of a sound whose fundamental is 200 Hz and whose spectrum contains the second and third harmonics. The amplitude of the fundamental is 12 v and the amplitude decreases by a factor of 2 for each successive higher harmonic.

6) The human auditory system is much more sensitive at 500 Hz then it is at 125 Hz. That is, a soft sound can be heard if it has a frequency of 500 Hz and it probably cannot be heard if it has a frequency of 125 Hz. A hearing scientist found that a 125-Hz sound presented at 50 dB SPL for 500 ms could not be detected, but yet when the duration of the sound was reduced to 8 ms it could be detected. Why might this happen?

7) Sketch the pulse train in the time domain for a pulse train with the amplitude spectrum shown below (assume that all components had 90° starting phases, and the amplitude of the pulse train can be any value).

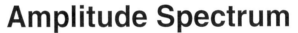

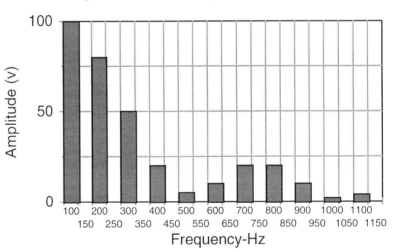

8) Knowing the difference between a rarefaction and a condensation transient, what change might you expect in the phase spectrum when going from a rarefaction to a condensation transient?

9) Two equal amplitude sinwaves are added. The difference in time between the major peaks of the waveform is 2 ms, and the difference in time between a minor and a major peak is 1 ms. What are the two frequencies and would such a waveform be likely to produce beats? Explain.

10) Given the amplitude spectrum of a sinusoidally amplitude-modulated tone shown below, what are the carrier and modulation frequencies of this SAM tone? What is the depth of modulation (m)?

Amplitude Spectrum

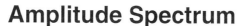
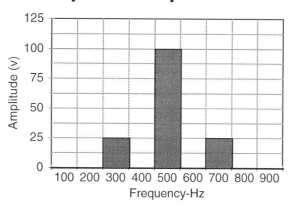

11) What is the difference between a tone that has a 50-Hz beat and one that is sinusoidally amplitude modulated at 50 Hz?

12) From the equation below, what is the carrier frequency, the modulation frequency, and the magnitude of the sinusoidal change in frequency? What might you hear if this sound was played?

$D(t) = 100\sin[2\pi((1500\ Hz)t)+(500Hz/25\ Hz)\sin(2\pi(25\ Hz)t)]$

13) If a sound's amplitude increases by a factor of two for each 10 ms of duration, and its frequency decreases by a factor of 2 for each 10 ms, what is the amplitude and frequency of the sound after 20 ms if its starting amplitude is 20 dB and its starting frequency is 16,000 Hz (amplitude is a pressure like term)? Draw a spectrogram (a three-dimensional bar graph) at 0, 10, and 20 ms.

14) A band of pink noise and a band of white noise are each centered at 1000 Hz and are 500 Hz wide. Each band of noise has the same total power. What would the total power of each noise be if the center frequency of each noise was increased to 2,000 Hz with a 1,000-Hz bandwidth?

15) Suppose a noise with a spectrum level of 25 dB makes it difficult to hear normal speech played in a background of the noise. How much total power would it take to produce a spectrum level of 25 dB if the noise bandwidth were 100 Hz and, then, what would the total power be in the bandwidth were 1,000 Hz?

16) On average the envelope frequency of a narrow band of noise is equal to 2/3 times the bandwidth of the noise. Suppose you wanted a noise with an average envelope frequency of 100 Hz and the lowest frequency in the band of noise was to be 500 Hz. What would the upper frequency be? Would the envelope of this narrow band of noise be periodic like that of an amplitude-modulated noise? Explain.

ADVANCED PROBLEMS

1) Using the equation below for a SAM tone with depth of modulation m, modulation frequency X1, and carrier frequency X2, expand the equation using the trigonometric identity shown below.

D(t) =A [1+$m$sin(X1)]sin(X2);

note that: sin(F1)sin(F2)= 1/2[cos(F1+F2) + cos(F1-F2)].

This expanded equation contains the carrier frequencies and sidebands and their amplitudes that were described for the spectrum of a SAM tone. Why?

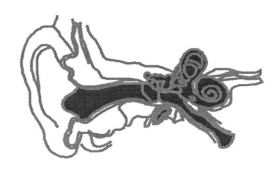

Answers for Problems for CHAPTER 4

1)

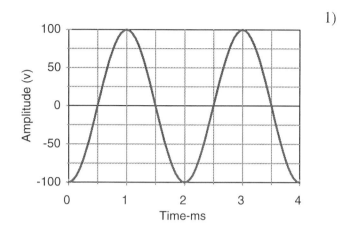

2)

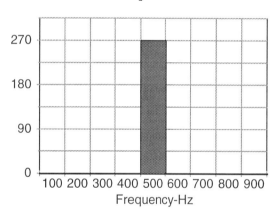

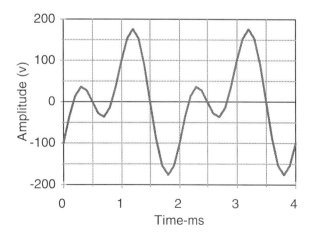

3)

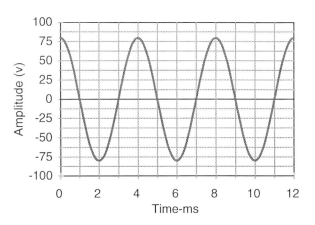

4) The time difference between the major peaks is 1.0 ms, suggesting a 1000-Hz tone. The time difference between the small peak and the big peak is 0.5 ms, suggesting a 2000-Hz tone.

5)

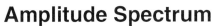
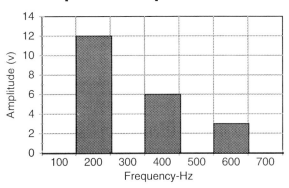

6) Perhaps the 8-ms, 125-Hz tone produced a spectrum with enough energy at 500 Hz that the listener detected this "energy splatter" at 500 Hz even though there was not enough energy at 125 Hz for detection. That is, at short durations a sinusoid has a large spectral region over which its energy is distributed.

7)

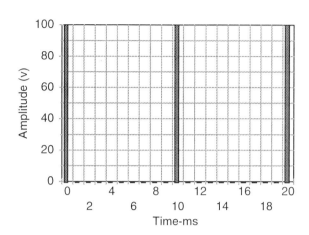

8) Since the difference between a rarefaction and a condensation transient is that one is positive going and the other negative going, there is a 180° phase difference between the two.

9) 2 ms would correspond to the period of 500 Hz and 1 ms to 1000 Hz, thus the two sinusoids might be 500 and 1000 Hz. These are so far apart in frequency that the two waveforms would probably not cause the perception of a beating tone.

10) Carrier frequency is 500 Hz, modulation frequency is 200 Hz, and the depth of modulation is 0.5 (m=0.5 or 100(m)/2 = 25, so m = 50/100 = 0.5).

11) A 50-Hz beat would be caused by a <u>two-tone complex</u>, where the two tones differed by 50 Hz, whereas a 50-Hz amplitude-modulated tone would be caused by a <u>three-tone complex</u>, with a carrier frequency and two sideband frequencies that each differed from the carrier frequency by 50 Hz.

12) Carrier frequency = 1,500 Hz, modulation frequency is 25 Hz, magnitude of the frequency change is 500 Hz.

13) After 20 ms the amplitude would be 32 dB, and the frequency would be 4,000 Hz. See figure below.

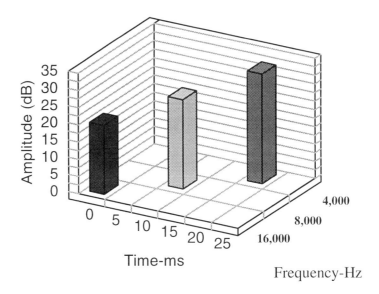

14) The total power for pink noise would not change at all, since total power for a pink noise remains the same as the center frequency changes and when the bandwidth is proportional to the center frequency. That is, a 1,000-Hz bandwidth at 2,000 Hz is proportional to a 1,000-Hz bandwidth at 500 Hz. The total power of the white noise would double, since the bandwidth doubled.

15) $TP_{dB} = No_{dB} + 10\log(BW)$; thus, $TP_{dB} = 25 + 10\log(100) = 25 + 20 = 45$ dB for the 100-Hz wide noise; and $TP_{dB} = 25 + 10\log(1,000) = 25 + 30 = 55$ dB for the 1000-Hz wide noise.

16) If envelope frequency = 2/3 bandwidth, then bandwidth=3/2(100)=150 Hz. Then, the upper frequency is 500 Hz + 150 Hz = 650 Hz. The envelope would not be periodic like that shown in Figure 14.7, but would be non-periodic like that shown in Figure 14.16. That is, only on average would the time between the major peaks in the envelope be 10 ms (i.e., the period of 100 Hz is 10 ms).

ADVANCED PROBLEMS

1) A $[1 + m \sin(X1)]\sin(X2) = A [\sin(X2) + m \sin(X1)\sin(X2)]$. Then,
   $m \sin(X1)\sin(X2) = m/2 [\cos(X1+X2) - \cos(X1-X2)]$, using the identity given in the problem. Thus,
   $A [1 + m\sin(X1)]\sin(X2) = A \sin(X2) + A(m/2) \cos(X1 + X2) + A(m/2) \cos(X1 - X2)$.
X2 is the carrier frequency with amplitude A, X1+X2 is the upper side band with amplitude A(m/2), and X1-X2 is the lower side band with amplitude A(m/2).

32

Chapter 5 - Sound Analysis

CD-ROM, Web Site, ASA Tapes: The CD-ROM and Web Site (*www.parmly.luc.edu/*) should be consulted.
ASA Tapes: Demonstration 33, Track 64,67. Demonstration 33 deals with distortion and nonlinearites.

Instructional Hints: A tuning fork is an excellent way to demonstrate concepts of resonance. Any simple flute-like instrument is helpful to discuss resonance in tubes.

Having students plot attenuation in dB/octave on both a log and a linear scale is a good way for them to appreciate the difference in these two scales and how the scales affect plotting.

Students need to understand that using a filter to estimate an amplitude spectrum only provides estimates of the relative levels of the frequency components and the spectral resolution is only as good as the filters bandwidths.

It is important that students understand that changes in the time-domain waveform cannot tell one if a system is linear or nonlinear.

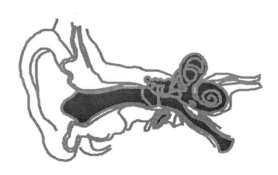

Chapter 5 - Suggested Problems for Students

1) A thin piece of metal is forced to vibrate at four different frequencies. The following rms amplitudes were measured:

At 500 Hz: 2 mm
At 750 Hz: 6 mm
At 1000 Hz: 4 mm
At 1250 Hz: 3.75 mm

What would be your best guess as to the resonant frequency of this piece of metal? Explain. Why should the amplitude of the forced vibration be kept constant as its frequency is changed when an object's resonant frequency is being measured?

2) An object has a resonant frequency of 1,200 Hz. Another similar object has the same stiffness but four times the mass, what is its resonant frequency?

3) Draw the filter shapes (usually called the transfer functions) for the following filters (draw the transfer function over a three-octave range from the filter's cutoff frequency and use an octave-frequency axis and a dB attenuation axis):

Filter Type	Cutoff Frequencies	Roll-off in dB/Octave
Low Pass	200 Hz	3
High Pass	10,000	6
Band Pass	1,000 and 2,000 Hz	10
Band Reject	2,000 and 8,000 Hz	12

[An octave-frequency axis is one in which each equal distant spacing is equal to a doubling (an octave) of the frequency--like Figure 5.2 in the Textbook]

4) Draw the low pass filter from problem 3) on a linear frequency axis and a linear attenuation axis. Assume that the level is measured in units of power or energy. Remember that each doubling or halving of power is 3 dB and that the level at 200 Hz is 10 units of power.

5) What are the 2nd and 5th harmonics and the 2nd and 5th octaves of 400 Hz?

6) Draw the output amplitude spectrum for the sound whose input amplitude spectrum is shown below after the sound is passed through a low pass filter with 400-Hz cutoff frequency and a 6-dB/octave roll-off.

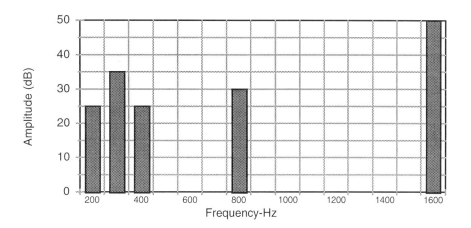

7) Shown below are the input and output amplitude spectra of a sound before and after it has been passed through a filter. Draw and describe this filter.

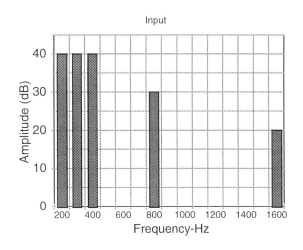
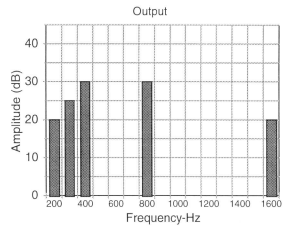

8) Which of the two time domain waveforms (A or B) shown below was likely to have been filtered by a low pass filter? Why?

A   B

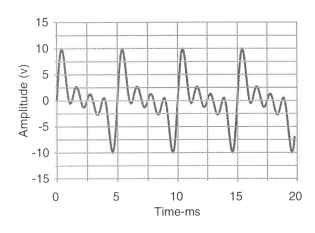
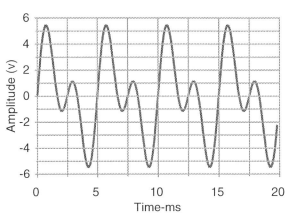

9) A common problem in building a place to test hearing is the fact that electrical current oscillates at about 60 Hz (so-called 60-cycle noise). How might you use a filter to reduce this 60-cycle noise on audio signals in your hearing facility? Be sure to specify the filter as fully as possible.

10) The outer ear canal (see Chapter 6 in the Textbook) is said to have a resonant frequency around 4,000-6,000 Hz because being a tube it produces standing waves. Suppose several tones of the same level were presented from a loudspeaker located near the ear canal and you were able to measure the levels in the outer ear canal. What would you predict would be the difference in the level measured for a 5,000-Hz tone as compared to that measured for a 100-Hz tone?

11) There are tiny bones (bones have mass and therefore inertia) in the middle ear (see Chapter 6 in the Textbook) that must vibrate for normal hearing to occur. Would these vibrating bones cause any potential loss of hearing sensitivity? If so, would it be for high or low frequencies and why? If not, why not?

12) Suppose that the vibration of the eardrum is to be measured. And, also suppose that a series of tones with the frequencies shown below are presented to the ear each at the same level and the resulting changes in level at the ear drum were measured? Using the concepts of Chapter 5, describe these changes:

500 Hz: 15 dB reduction
1,000 Hz: no reduction
2,000 Hz: 15 dB increase
4,000 Hz: no reduction
8,000 Hz: 15 dB reduction
16,000 Hz: 30 dB reduction

13) When your radio is turned up too loud it distorts the sound because the amplifier in the radio is acting nonlinearly. Suppose the sound being played is the sum of two equal amplitude sinusoids with frequencies of 350 and 900 Hz, and suppose the order of the nonlinearity of the radio is 3 (m and n = 3). Describe all of the sound frequencies that the radio would produce. Which are harmonic tones, combination tones, summation tones, and difference tones?

14) The human auditory system is very sensitive to the cubic-difference tone. When a two-tone waveform (frequencies of F1 and F2) is played the cubic difference tone has the frequency of 2F1-F2, which is twice the frequency of the higher tone (F2) minus the frequency of the lower tone (F1). If F1 is 1,200 Hz, what would F2 have to be in order for a person to hear a 600-Hz cubic difference tone? What is the ratio of F1 to F2?

15) A computer music person generates a sound on a synthesizer that consists of a fundamental frequency and its 12 upper harmonics. When she plays it, it doesn't sound correct to her. Her boss says it is because the loudspeaker has filtered the wave and not all of the harmonics are coming through at the amplitudes she programmed for them. Her friend says that the amplifier may be nonlinear and, therefore, it is distorting the sound. She decides to test the entire system (synthesizer, amplifier, and loudspeaker) by playing a series of sinwaves through the entire system. She discovered that both her boss and her friend were correct; there was some lowpass filtering and some nonlinearity. What must have she measured in terms of changes from the input sinwaves to output sinwaves of her system?

ADVANCED PROBLEMS

1) We will find that the auditory system performs a type of operation that is like bandpass filtering, such that the bandpass filters have approximately equal Q. If the Q of a filter centered at 1,000 Hz is 10, what is the bandwidth of a filter centered at 8,000 Hz?

2) Show why equation A.19 in Appendix A, does not follow the superposition requirement.

3) If $x(t)=\sin(2\pi ft)$, then show what happens when, $y(t)=x(t) + x(t)^2$. That is, show how the squaring operation produces the second harmonic (2f) of f. What are the amplitude and phase of the harmonic component relative to those for the fundamental component?[hint: $\sin(x)\sin(x) = 1/2(1-\cos2a)$]

Answers for Problems for CHAPTER 5

1) Since the greatest amplitude was at 750 Hz, this would be the best guess for the resonant frequency. If the amplitude of the forced vibration is not kept fixed, then it is difficult to know if a change in amplitude of the object being vibrated is due to resonance or the driving amplitude.

2) Since fr=[$\sqrt{}$ (s/m)]/2π, and the mass (m) is increased by a factor of four, the frequency would decrease by a factor of 2 ($\sqrt{}$ 4), that is, it would be 600 Hz.

3)

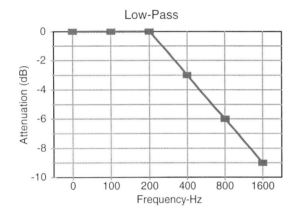
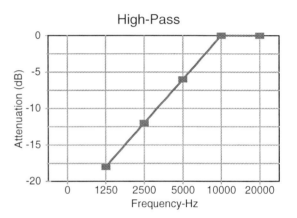
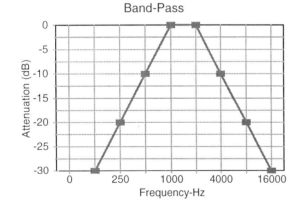
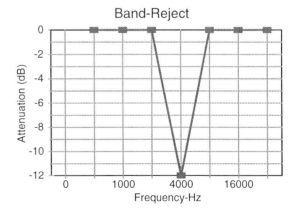

4)

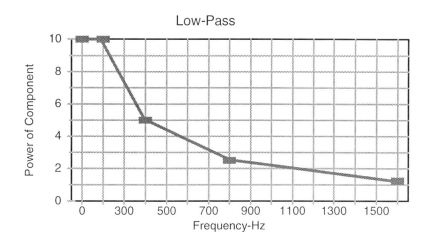

5) The 2nd harmonic of 400 Hz is 800 Hz, 5th harmonic is 2000 Hz, first octave is 800 Hz, and the 5th octave is 12,800 Hz.

6)

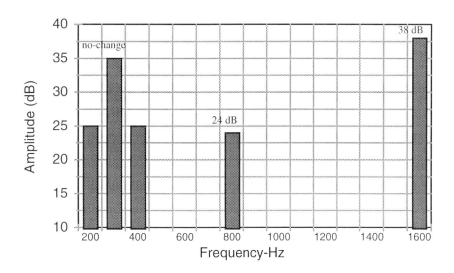

7)

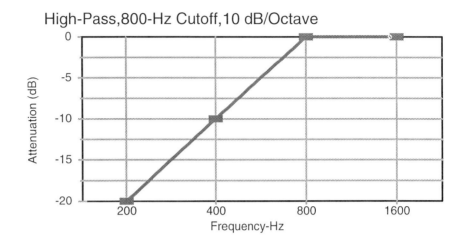

High-Pass,800-Hz Cutoff,10 dB/Octave

8) The waveform in panel B, since its periods of vibration are lower than those of A, indicating the A has higher frequencies than B.

9) Use either a highpass filter with a cutoff just above 60 Hz and with a steep rolloff, or a band-reject filter with 60 Hz being in the middle of the rejection band of the filter (again a steep rolloff would be advantageous).

10) Sounds with frequencies at 5,000 Hz would probably have greater amplitude than those near 100 Hz, since the sounds near 5,000 Hz would be increased by the resonance properties of the outer ear canal.

11) Since bones have mass they would act as lowpass filters and, thus, might reduce the sensitivity for hearing high-frequency sounds. (We will learn that these middle-ear bones are the lightest bones in the body, which helps to reduce the amount of lowpass filtering they might introduce.)

12) The shape of the curve relating vibration to frequency shows a peak at 2,000 Hz. This might indicate that the eardrum has a resonance frequency at or near 2,000 Hz, thus increasing the level of vibration for sounds of this frequency.

13) F_1=350 Hz   (negative frequencies are not included)
     F_2=900 Hz
     $2F_1$=700 Hz   : Harmonics
     $2F_2$=1,800 Hz   : Harmonics
     $3F_1$=1,050 Hz   : Harmonics
     $3F_2$=2,700 Hz   : Harmonics

F1+F2=1,250 Hz   :   Combination tones/summation tones
F1+2F2=2,150 Hz   :   Combination tones/summation tones
F1+3F2=3,050 Hz   :   Combination tones/summation tones
2F1+F2=1,600 Hz   :   Combination tones/summation tones
2F1+2F2=2,500 Hz :   Combination tones/summation tones
2F1+3F2=3,400 Hz :   Combination tones/summation tones
3F1+F2=1,950 Hz   :   Combination tones/summation tones
3F1+2F2=2,850 Hz :   Combination tones/summation tones
3F1+3F2=3,750 Hz :   Combination tones/summation tones
F2-F1=550 Hz   :   Combination tones/difference tones
F2-2F1=150   :   Combination tones/difference tones
2F2-F1= 1,550 Hz :   Combination tones/difference tones
2F2-2F1=1,100 Hz :   Combination tones/difference tones
2F2-3F1=750 Hz   :   Combination tones/difference tones
3F2-F1=2,350 Hz   :   Combination tones/difference tones
3F2-2F1=2,000 Hz :   Combination tones/difference tones
3F2-3F1=1,650 Hz :   Combination tones/difference tones

14) 600 Hz = 2(1,200 Hz) - F2; F2= 2,400 - 600 = 1,800 Hz. F1/F2 = 1,200/1,800 = 2/3.

15) If the loudspeaker acted as a low pass filter, then the high-frequency components of the output would be attenuated relative to the low-frequency components (and these high-frequencies components may also undergo a phase shift relative to the low-frequency components). If in addition to lowpass filtering, the system was nonlinear, then frequency components would exist at the output that were not in the input. These new frequency components would be harmonics and combination tones of the input frequencies.

ADVANCED PROBLEMS

1) Q=CF/BW, BW = CF/Q, so BW at 8,000 Hz = 8,000/10 = 800 Hz, where CF is center frequency and BW is bandwidth.

2) If $y(t) = x(t) + x^2(t)$, and $x(t) = \sin(2\pi f1t)+\sin(2\pi f2t)$; then $y(t) = [\sin(2\pi f1t)+\sin(2\pi f2t)] + [\sin(2\pi f1t)+\sin(2\pi f2t)]^2$ does not equal $[\sin(2\pi f1t)]+[\sin(2\pi f1t)]^2+ [\sin(2\pi f2t)]+[\sin(2\pi f2t)]^2$, which is what needs to exist for superposition to hold.

3) $y(t)=x(t) + x(t)^2 = \sin(2\pi ft) + \sin(2\pi ft)^2 = \sin(2\pi ft) + \sin(2\pi ft)\sin(2\pi ft) =$
$\sin(2\pi ft) + ½ + ½ \cos(2\pi 2ft)$. So f and $2f$ (the harmonic of f) are present. The level of the harmonic component ($2f$) is ½ that of the fundamental component (f), and the phase of the harmonic component differs by 90° from that of the fundamental component (due to the 90° phase difference between the sin and cos functions).

41

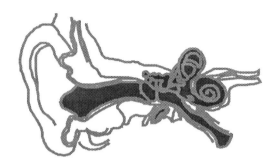

Chapter 6 - The Outer and Middle Ears

CD-ROM, Web Site, ASA Tapes: The CD-ROM and Web Site (*www.parmly.luc.edu/*) should be consulted.

Instructional Hints: With the change in topics from physics and engineering for chapters 1-5 to biology for chapters 6-9, the students may need some time to adjust. Appendix E might help in that adjustment. The students need to be reminded that while much of the discussion in chapters 6-9 is biological, all of the material covered in the first five chapters will be used extensively in discussing auditory physiology.

The instructor should note that many of the problems for this section cover "practical" uses of the concepts covered in the Textbook. These uses can also help describe outer and middle ear anatomy and physiology.

It is probably a good idea to have students use a ruler marked in millimeters so that they can appreciate the very small sizes of the outer and middle ear structures.

Changes in impedance from air to fluids can be explained by having students think about the ease with which they can move their hands through air as opposed to water.

Problems 8-10 in the next section deal with HRTF measurement, the advanced students need to realize that in addition to the two spectra described in the problem, the spectrum of the transfer function of the microphone and/or canal measurement tube would also have to be included in the final measurement of the HRTF.

Another, surgical procedure that use to be performed, a fenestration operation, helps explain middle ear function. The fenestration operation was designed to deal with abnormal osscicular chains. One outcome of the fenestration procedure was that airborne sound would impinge upon both the round and oval windows, although more on the oval window. As a result the operation did not restore hearing to anywhere near normal levels. When both windows are stimulated the pressure difference across the basilar membrane is reduced, leading to reduced basilar membrane motion.

Chapter 6 - Suggested Problems for Students

1) At the end of this chapter are several sample drawings that can be used to test students about the anatomy of the outer and middle ears.

2) Which of the gross divisions of the auditory system contain neural elements?

3) Which structure of the middle ear is the biggest and which is the smallest?

4) What connects the tympanic membrane to the inner ear?

5) When you have a cold and travel in an airplane, you might experience pain in your "ears" as the pressure in the cabin changes suddenly. As the plane ascends, air pressure can decrease. Similar pain is often experienced when one dives underwater, when one has a cold. The further one dives underwater, the greater the air pressure. Having a cold blocks the nasal passages. Also, undue stretching of the tympanic membrane causes pain. Why would having a cold cause an "earache" when the pressure changes as described above?

6) Why might the bones, muscles, and ligaments of the middle ear be among the lightest in the entire body?

7) Why do the structures of the outer ear (e.g., the pinna) attenuate the amplitudes of tones with high, but not low, frequencies? (hint: recall from Chapter 3 the idea of a sound shadow and the relationship between the size of an object and a sound's wavelength)

Problems 8-10: The following table provides the input spectra for a sound source and the spectra measured near the tympanic membrane.

	Input Spectra		Spectra at the Tympanic Membrane			
			Left Ear		Right Ear	
Freq.	Amplitude	Phase	Amplitude	Phase	Amplitude	Phase
(Hz)	(dB)	(degs)	(dB)	(degs)	(dB)	(degs)
250	50	0	45	36	35	126
500	50	0	45	36	35	216
1,000	50	0	55	45	40	405
2,000	50	0	50	45	35	765
3,000	55	0	40	90	20	1,170
4,000	60	0	35	180	15	1,620
5,000	65	45	25	135	0	1,935
8,000	70	90	40	90	0	2,970

8) Provide a Table describing the HRTF amplitudes for each ear.

9) What are the interaural time differences at each test frequency? (Hint: time=phase x period/360°; each 360° of phase represents one period of the sinwave)

10) For the conditions shown for Problems 8 and 9, on what side of the head was the input sound source located? Explain.

11) A stapedechtomy is an operation in which the ossicular chain may be removed and replaced by a single "strut" that connects the tympanic membrane to the oval window of the inner ear. By removing the ossicular chain the leverage action of the ossicular chain and the size difference between the manubrium and the footplate of the stapes can be lost. How many decibels of hearing loss might a person have after this type of stapedechtomy? Explain your answer.

12) Assume that the fluids of the inner ear are about 25 times more difficult to move than air and that this would result in the same proportional decrease in inner ear pressure relative to that in air. Speech contains frequencies primarily in the range from 300 to 3,000 Hz. Given the transfer function of the middle ear, there is very little loss of pressure between air and the fluids of the inner ear over the speech-frequency range. That is, for speech the structures of the inner ear move without much loss of pressure demonstrating an impedance match between air and the inner-ear fluids over this frequency range. Use the appropriate figure of the Textbook and calculations to explain why this is true.

13) When you complained to the manager of a movie theater that the sounds are dangerously loud, he responds by saying that you should not worry because your middle ear muscles protect you against hearing loss. What aspects of middle ear muscle function indicate that they might not protect you from hearing damage caused by a wide variety of intense movie sounds?

14) Placing a vibrating device on the forehead leads to audible sound in that the sound travels through the bones and directly vibrates the fluids of the inner ear. Thus, this form of hearing is called bone conduction and does not involve the middle ear structures. Consider two people with hearing loss: Person A has abnormal hearing when sounds are presented to the ears over headphones, but person A hears the same as normal-hearing people when they are stimulated by placing a vibrator on the forehead. Person B has abnormal hearing when sounds are presented over headphones and when the bone vibrator is used. One person appears to have a damaged ossicular chain, and the other person is experiencing some other difficulty. Which person is which? Explain.

15) Suppose an electroacoustic impedance bridge is used to measure middle ear function in a patient with a hearing loss and both low-frequency and high-frequency probe tones are used. Suppose that the bridge measures normal responses for the low-frequency probe but the measures are abnormal for the high-frequency probe. What kind of abnormality might this indicate?

ADVANCED PROBLEMS

1) In the Summary of Outer and Middle Ear Measures given at the end of Chapter 6 in the Textbook, it is pointed out that the tympanic membrane breaks when it is exposed to a pressure of 1.61×10^6 dynes/cm^2. If the threshold for hearing sounds is 0.0002 dynes/cm^2)(20 μPa = 0.0002 dynes/cm^2), how many decibels above threshold (i.e., dB SPL) will cause the tympanic membrane to break?

2) At 65 dB SPL the tympanic membrane is displaced 5 Å (from the Summary of Outer and Middle Ear Measures given at the end of Chapter 6 in the Textbook). Assuming that the measurements were linear, what would be the displacement of the tympanic membrane at the threshold for hearing (i.e., at 0 dB SPL)? Note that the diameter of a hydrogen atom is about 2.4 Å.

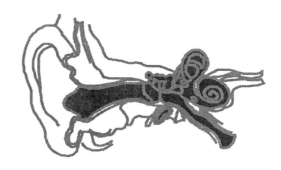

Answers for Problems for CHAPTER 6

2) The inner ear and the central auditory nervous system as depicted in Fig. 6.1 of the Textbook contain neural elements.

3) The malleus is the largest bone and the stapes is the smallest bone.

4) The ossicles connect the tympanic membrane to the oval window of the inner ear.

5) A cold would block the nasal passages. The eustachian tube connects to the nasal passages to allow air pressure to equalize across the tympanic membrane. If this passage from the middle ear to the eustachian tube to the nasal passages is blocked, then as pressure on the outside of the tympanic membrane changes (decreases as one goes up in an airplane or increases as one dives underwater), the pressure changes cannot be equalized. The opposite happens under water; the deeper one goes, the greater the pressure that cannot be equalized. Hence, the tympanic membrane will be stretched abnormally (it will be pushed in for the water example and pulled out for the airplane example). This stretching may cause pain.

6) These structures of the middle ear must move in response to sound. If they were massive then they would be difficult to move and would decrease hearing sensitivity. According to the discussions of Chapter 5 of the Textbook, objects with mass act as lowpass filters. The heavier the mass, the lower the cutoff frequency. Thus, light structures mean high cutoff frequencies, so that hearing can take place at high frequencies.

7) The ability of an object to attenuate (block) a sound depends on the relationship between the wavelength of the sound wave and the size of the object (see Chapter 3 in the Textbook). If the wavelength is large relative to the size of the object, then there is little attenuation. Since most of the structures of the outer ear are small, they would only block (attenuate) sounds with short wavelengths. High-frequency sounds have short wavelengths, and thus, these small outer ear structures would only attenuate high-frequency sounds.

8) To construct the table of the HRTF amplitudes, the amplitudes measured at the input are subtracted from those measured at the tympanic membrane and are therefore expressed as values of attenuation (negative values) or gain (positive values).

Thus:

Freq. (Hz)	Left Ear Amplitude (dB)	Right Ear Amplitude (dB)
250	45-50=**-5**	35-50=**-15**
500	45-50=**-5**	35-50=**-15**
1,000	55-50=**+5**	40-50=**-10**
2,000	50-50=**0**	35-50=**-15**
3,000	40-55=**-15**	20-55=**-35**
4,000	35-60=**-25**	15-60=**-45**
5,000	25-65=**-40**	0-65=**-65**
8,000	40-70=**-30**	0-70=**-70**

9) The phase difference between the left and right ears is determined independent of the phase of the input, since the input phase is a constant added to the phase measurements obtained at both ears. Hence, subtracting the phases at the left ear from those at the right ear yields:

Freq. (Hz)	Period (ms)	Interaural Phase Difference (degs)	Interaural Time Difference (ms)
250	4	126-36=90	90*4/360=1 ms
500	2	216-36=180	180*2/360=1 ms
1,000	1	405-45=360	360*1/360=1 ms
2,000	0.5	765-45=720	720*0.5/360=1 ms
3,000	0.33	1,170-90=1,080	1,080*0.33/360=1 ms
4,000	0.25	1,620-180=1,440	1,440*0.25/360=1 ms
5,000	0.2	1,935-135=1,800	1,800*0.2/360=1 ms
8,000	0.125	2,970-90=2,880	2,800*0.125/360= 1 ms

Thus, there is a constant interaural time difference of 1 ms, indicating that it took 1 ms for the sound to travel from the left to the right ear.

10) The sound must be on the left side of the head since the amplitudes are lower on the right side and the sound is delayed at the right ear relative to that at the left ear.

11) The gain due to the lever action is a factor of 1.3 and that of the area difference is a factor of 17. Thus, 1.3*17= 22.1 increase with an intact ossicular chain. Thus, without an intact ossicular chain, a maximum hearing loss of a factor of 22.1 might occur. 20*log(22.1) is 26.9 dB, which is the decibel loss that might occur.

48

12) The fluids of the inner ear are 25 times more difficult to move which could produce about a 28 dB loss (20*log(25)=27.96 dB). But according to Fig. 6.8 the middle ear provides about a 25-30 dB gain in the region of 500 to 3000 Hz. Thus, in this frequency region the gain provided by the middle ear cancels the loss caused by the difference in the density of the fluids.

13) The middle ear muscles are slow acting and they provide the most protection at low frequencies. Thus, any sounds that occur with sudden onsets and that are mainly high frequencies may not be attenuated a great deal by the middle ear muscles, even if the sound levels are high.

14) Person A may have a damaged ossicular chain. Since sound seems to vibrate the inner ear when the middle ear is bypassed, it is unlikely that the inner ear is damaged. When sound has to go through the middle ear, as it does for sound delivered over headphones, then this person experiences a hearing loss. Person B probably has something wrong with the inner ear or central auditory nervous system, since sounds that get to the inner ear are difficult to hear no matter how the vibrations arrived at the inner ear.

15) An abnormal response at high frequencies would indicate a type of mass-reactance problem. Since the middle ears ossicles (bones) are the most massive structures in the middle ear, an impedance abnormality at high frequencies might indicate a problem with the ossicles.

ADVANCED PROBLEMS

1) 0.0002 dynes/cm^2 is 2 X 10^{-4} dynes/cm^2. So, 1.61 X 10^6 dynes/cm^2 is 1.61/2 X 10^{10} = 0.805 X 10^{10} =8.05 X 10^9 times greater pressure than the pressure of 2 X 10^{-4} dynes/cm^2. 20*log(8.05X10^9) = 20*log(8.05)+20*log(10^9)=18.1 + 180=198.1 dB. So a sound at 198 dB SPL could rupture the tympanic membrane.

2) 65 dB is a factor of 1778.3 greater than 0 dB ($10^{65/20}$=1778.23) in pressure. Pressure is proportional to displacement squared (see Chapter 3 in the Textbook). Thus, the square root of 1778 is about 42. Therefore, at threshold (0 dB SPL) the movement (displacement) of the tympanic membrane is 5/42 = 0.11 $\overset{0}{A}$, which is smaller than the diameter of a hydrogen atom.

49

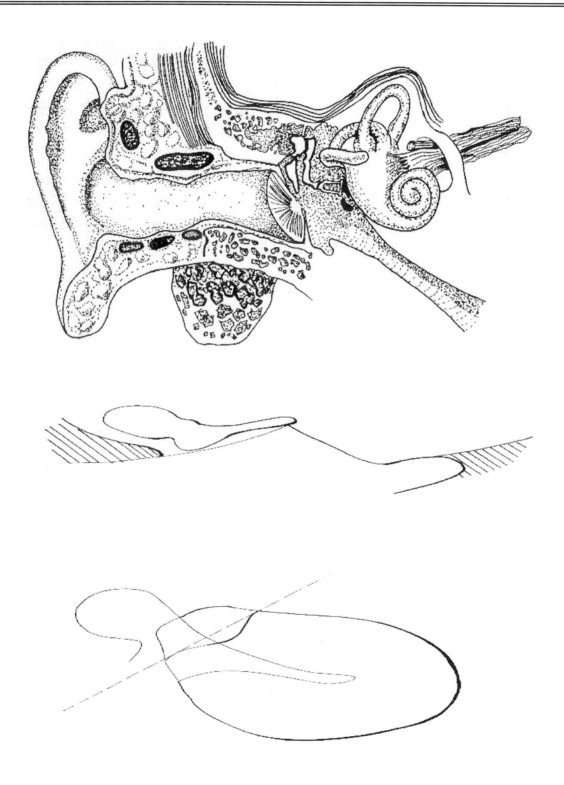

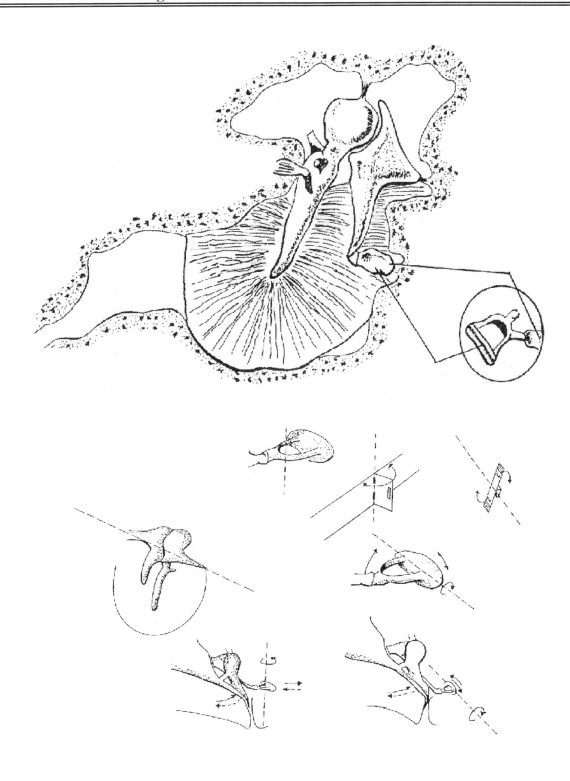

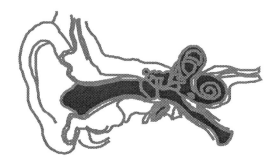

Chapter 7 - Structure of the Inner Ear and Its Mechanical Response

CD-ROM, Web Site, ASA Tapes: The CD-ROM and Web Site (*www.parmly.luc.edu/*) should be consulted.

Instructional Hints: Scala media is like an inner tube with an outer tube. The space between the inner and outer tubes is the scala vestibuli (above) and scala tympani (below). These tubes are wrapped around an axis (the modiolus) as it is coiled.

Using a long rope (about 3 meters long) may be useful to demonstrate the traveling wave. First, have a student hold one end as you vibrate the other end of the rope. You should be able to establish a standing wave. You can explain that the standing wave gets established because the vibration reflects off the hand holding the other end of the rope and reinforces and cancels the wave motion coming from the end that is being vibrated. However, the basilar membrane is not attached at its end (the helicotrema). Thus, have the student let go of the rope and let it lie on the floor. Now, vibrate the rope as fast as you can. With any luck only the part of the rope near your moving hand will vibrate-- the end of the rope will be nearly still. Thus, high frequencies vibrate only near the vibrating object (i.e., the base). Now vibrate the rope slowly. The rope should move (travel) toward your hand. This is, therefore, a traveling wave because the rope is unattached at the end. With the low-frequency movement of the rope there is vibration all along the rope. If you are very careful at vibrating the rope at the proper low frequency, you can get a little more displacement toward the end of the rope than near your moving hand. While the basilar membrane does not actually move like the rope, the demonstration captures many properties of the cochlear traveling wave. In addition to the basilar membrane not having a point at the end for reflections, the changes in the width and tension of the membrane from base to apex also help establish the traveling wave motion.

To make a point about sensory coding, you can point out that all one has to do is to note which end of the rope is vibrating to figure out the frequency of vibration. That is, where the vibration occurs codes for frequency; high frequencies at the base and low frequencies at the apex.

When discussing the nonlinearity of basilar membrane motion, the material in Chapter 16 of the textbook might be consulted, especially the section on Relationship Between Inner Ear Damage and Hearing Loss.

Chapter 7 - Suggested Problems for Students

1) At the end of this chapter are several sample drawings that can be used to test students about the anatomy of the inner ear.

2) In addition to hearing, what other sense is served by the inner ear?

3) A cross-section of the cochlea is like a tube divided into three sections. What are these three sections; which one contains the sensory cells that transduce vibration into neural impulses?

4) What are the sensory cells and where does each lie in relationship to the modiolus and the stria vascularis?

5) The sensory cells lie between which two membranes? What two membranes mark the boundary of scala media.

6) What are the "hair-like" structures that give the hair cells their name?

7) The size of the cochlea and that of the basilar membrane differs from base to apex. What are the general differences of the size of each between the base and apex?

8) What structure supplies the basic metabolic energy for the cochlea?

9) What is the overall function of the cochlea?

10) Why is the cochlea often called a frequency analyzer?

11) You observe that the motion of the basilar membrane is maximal 30 mm from the base. If the basilar membrane responds to frequencies over the range from 50 to 25,000 Hz, which of the following tones was most likely the stimulating tone? A tone with a frequency of 20,000 Hz, 10,000 Hz, or 250 Hz? Why?

12) A particular stimulus causes three places of maximal displacement of basilar-membrane motion? Is this a mistake? If not, what kind of stimulus might explain this type of response? Explain.

13) Define each of the following: traveling wave, instantaneous basilar membrane pattern, envelope of the traveling wave.

14) If it takes 4 ms for the traveling wave to travel from the base to the apex, what would the phase shift be for a 1,000-Hz tone measured at the apex? (Remember that every 360° of phase shift is equal to one period.) What would this phase shift be for a 125-Hz tone?

Problems 15-18: Tabled below are hypothetical data (displacement in micrometers) obtained from one location on the basilar membrane for tones of different frequencies and levels.

Tonal Frequency (Hz)	Level of the Tone (in dB SPL)					
	10	20	30	40	50	60
2,000	5	10	15	20	23	24
3,000	10	15	20	25	28	30
4,000	20	25	30	35	38	40
5,000	15	20	25	30	33	35
6,000	10	15	20	25	29	31
7,000	1	6	10	15	18	20
8,000	0	0	1	10	15	20

15) At 40 dB SPL, plot displacement in micrometers as a function of frequency.

16) Plot the isosensitivity function for 20 micrometers. That is, for each frequency plot the level of the tone required to achieve 20 micrometers of basilar membrane displacement.

17) What frequency is this place on the basilar membrane responding best to? If the basilar membrane response to frequencies from 50 to 25,000 Hz, is this place on the basilar membrane nearer the base, middle, or apex?

18) Each plot (Problems 15 and 16) reflects a bandpass characteristic of cochlear action. What is the center frequency of this filter and what are the approximate high- and low-frequency roll offs (in dB/Octave)?

19) The following basilar membrane measurements were made:

Sound Level (dB SPL)	Velocity (micormeters/sec)	
	Stimulus A	Stimulus B
20		10
40		100
60	10	333
80	100	1,000
100	1,000	10,000

Plot these data for both stimuli A and B as velocity versus sound level, with a linear x-axis and a logarithmic y-axis. A logarithmic y-axis is established such that each equal distance on the axis is a factor of 10. So the distance from 10 to 100 is the same as that from 100 to 1,000 and that from 1000 to 10,000. The number 333 would be half way between 100 and 1,000.

Which stimulus (A or B) shows a linear input-output response? Over what sound level range is the nonlinear input-output function compressive?

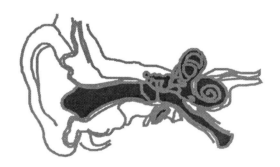

Answers for Problems for CHAPTER 7

2) The sense of balance or the vestibular system is served by the inner ear.

3) The three sections or scala are (from top to bottom): scala vestibuli, scala media, scala tympani; and the scala media contains the sensory and supporting cells.

4) The sensory cells are the inner and outer haircells. The inner haircells lie closest to the modiolus and the outer haircells closest to the stria vascularis.

5) Haircells lie between the basilar and tectorial membranes. The bottom border of scala media is basilar membrane and the top border is Reissner's membrane.

6) The hair-like structures are the stereocilia (or cilia).

7) Basilar membrane is wider at the apex than at the base, while the cochlea becomes smaller from base to apex.

8) The stria vascularis provides the blood supply and, thus, the metabolic energy for the cochlea.

9) The cochlea transduces sound vibrations (that cause vibration of the fluids and the structures of the inner ear) into neural signals; these neural signals code for the frequency, intensity, and phase of the sound.

10) The cochlea is called a "frequency analyzer" because the action of the traveling wave decomposes a complex vibration into a frequency specific pattern of vibration distributed along the cochlea such that high frequencies cause maximal basilar membrane vibration at the base and low frequencies cause maximal vibration at the apex.

11) Since the basilar membrane is only about 35 mm long, 30 mm must be close to the apex; thus, maximal vibration would be caused by a low-frequency sound. In this case this would be the 250-Hz tone.

12) It is not a mistake for there to be multiple peaks in the envelope of basilar membrane vibration. Such multiple peaks could indicate that the complex sound has several frequencies each with about equal amplitude. So three peaks could be a caused by a complex sound with three sinwaves.

13) The traveling wave is the motion of the basilar membrane in which the location of maximal vibration is frequency dependent. The instantaneous basilar membrane pattern is the position of the basilar membrane at one instant in time. The envelope of the traveling wave is an estimate of the overall pattern of basilar membrane vibration over a fairly long period of time.

14) A 1,000-Hz tone has a 1-ms period. 4 ms is thus 4 periods and with each period being 360°, the phase at the apex would be 1440° (4x360°). For a 125-Hz tone with an 8-ms period, 4 ms is one half a period or 180°.

15)

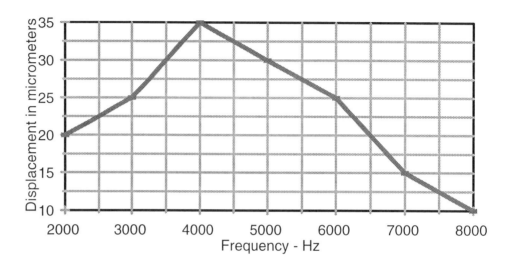

16)

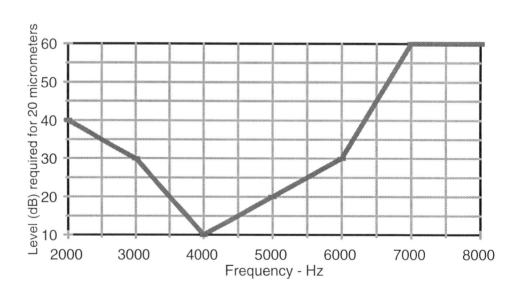

17) This location along the basilar membrane is responding best to 4,000 Hz. This place would be near the middle or the apex side of the middle of the cochlear partition.

18) If these recordings were like a bandpass filter the center frequency would be 4,000 Hz. Since the level in Figure 16 changes by 30 dB from 4,000 to 2,000 Hz (one octave), the roll off on the low-frequency side is 30 dB/octave. The level changes by 50 dB from 4,000 to 8,000 Hz (one octave), so the roll off is 50 dB/octave on the high-frequency side.

19) Stimulus A shows the linear input-output relationship.

Stimulus B shows a compressive non-linearity from 40 to 80 dB SPL

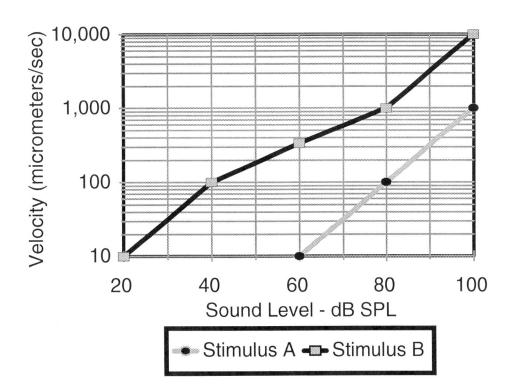

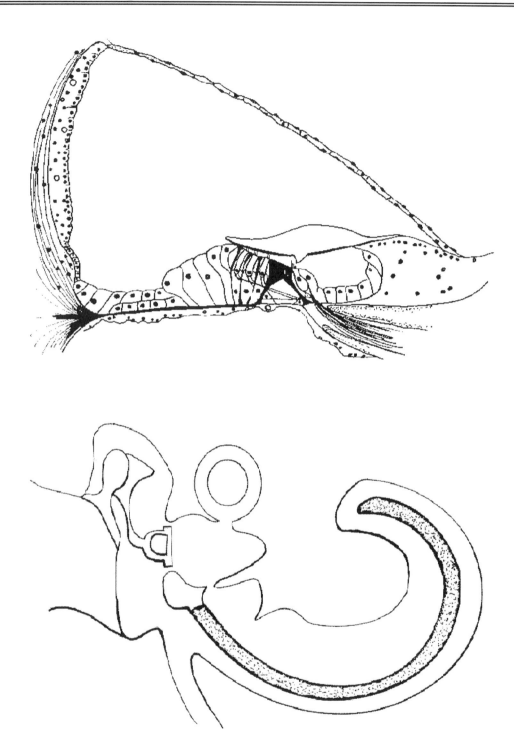

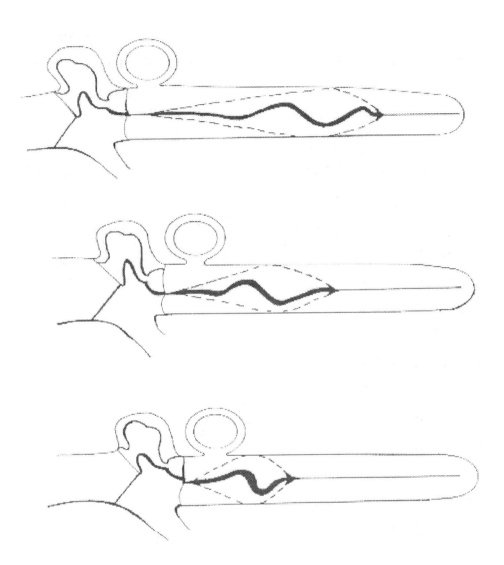

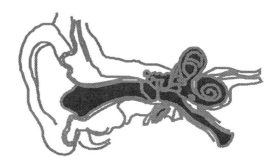

Chapter 8 - Peripheral Auditory Nervous System and Haircells

CD-ROM, Web Site, ASA Tapes: The CD-ROM and Web Site (*www.parmly.luc.edu/*) should be consulted.

Instructional Hints: It is often helpful to use a battery to light a light bulb to provide simple demonstrations about currents, potential differences, and voltages. It is important that students appreciate the fact that current flows from one point to another, and thus, a reference electrode at a neutral electrical site is required to measure current flow.

To get a "feel" for *shearing forces*, model the two membranes with your hands. Put your right hand palm up, and place your left hand on it palm down. Slide your right hand forward so that the fingers of the fight hand extend about 1/2 inch farther than those of the left. Now, keeping your palms still and your fingers stiff, move the fingers of both hands up and down simultaneously, and you can feel the shearing forces in your fingers.

The study of the inner ear and its mechanical and neural function is rapidly changing. The issue of how the outer haircell's motility operates in a living animal is still largely unknown. Thus, the exact way in which outer haircell function aids in sound transduction is still being debated. As a result, concepts like feedback, the cochlear amplifier, and the connection between outer haircell motility and auditory emissions are all likely to undergo considerable changes in the next few years.

It is probably worth pointing out to students that a great deal of skill is required to perform many of the experiments that form the basis of the material in this chapter. Excising haircells, making intercellular recordings from haircells, manipulating stereocilia, etc. are very difficult techniques that require considerable skill and experience. All of these involve dealing with tissue that is far from that which occurs in the normal-behaving animal. Thus, some caution is also necessary in interpreting the data from these in vitro experiments to the in vivo state. This is especially true, given how vulnerable the inner ear is to damage.

Much of the material in Chapter 16 of the textbook and of this workbook is relevant to understanding the inner ear. A great deal of the knowledge of inner ear function has been obtained from experiments in which the inner ear is damaged in one way or the other. Some of this material is presented in Chapter 16, The Abnormal Auditory System.

Chapter 8 - Suggested Problems for Students

1) At the end of this chapter are two sample drawings that can be used to test students about the anatomy of the inner ear and haircells.

2) Name the four electrical potentials that can be measured within the cochlea.

3) The figure below represents electrical measurements made in the cochlea. The duration of stimulation was 20 ms. The potential on top is shown as the negative of the actual measured response (i.e., actual negative potentials are plotted as positive and actual positive potentials as negative). What potential is probably shown on top? Which two potentials are represented by the bottom potential? What was the probable frequency of stimulation? Where (near the base or apex) were these measurements most likely made? Explain.

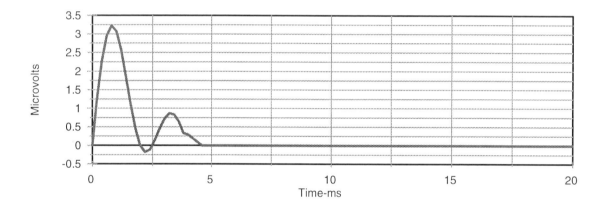

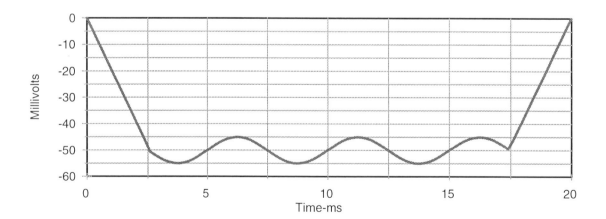

4) How are these cochlear potentials measured?

5) Which potential is a neural potential and not a true cochlear potential?

6) The shearing action which causes *haircell stereocilia* to bend is caused by the differential movement between which two membranes?

7) Which haircells display motile responses when stimulated?

8) What function might haircell motility play in the neural transduction of sound vibration into neural impulses?

9) Name and describe the three types of *otoacoustic emissions*.

10) How might *otoacoustic emissions* and *haircell motility* be related?

11) List the four types of afferent auditory nerve fibers and describe how each type innervates haircells.

12) Which type of afferent fiber is most likely carrying most of the information about sound to the central nervous system and which type of haircell do these fibers innervate?

13) How are the nerve fibers organized within the VIII nerve?

14) What is the functional difference between efferent and afferent nerve fibers?

15) How does the innervation of the efferent fibers differ between inner and outer haircells?

16) What is the probable relationship between efferent fibers and otoacoustic emissions?

17) Describe the key steps that take place from the motion of the stapes to neural impulses in an auditory nerve.

ADVANCED PROBLEMS

1) Why would the *extratympanic* measurement of the *AP* be less sensitive than the *transtympanic* measurement?

2) Why are acoustic emissions an attractive possibility as a measure of hearing in infants?

Answers for Problems for CHAPTER 8

2) The four inner ear electrical potentials are: the *cochlear microphonic, summating potential, resting potential*, and the *action potential* (while recorded in the inner ear the AP is a neural response and not a true cochlear potential).

3) The top "potential" is probably the action potential. The bottom potential shows both the DC shift of the *summating potential* and the oscillation of the *cochlear microphonic*. The *cochlear microphonic* part of the bottom trace has a period of 5 ms, which would indicate a 200-Hz tone was probably the stimulating tone. A 200-Hz tone would be best recorded near the apex.

4) Cochlear potentials are best measured with the differential electrode technique in which a recording electrode is placed in the inner ear in different turns of the cochlea to measure the potentials at different places along the cochlear partition.

5) The *Action Potential*, while measured in the inner ear, is not a true cochlear potential, but represents the synchronous firing of many auditory nerve fibers.

6) The shear is between *basilar* and *tectorial* membranes.

7) Only outer haircells demonstrate motility.

8) Outer haircell motility seems to be important to maintain the high sensitivity of inner haircells and their great frequency selectivity. The outer haircells may help control the coupling between the basilar and tectorial membranes as a means to most efficiently stimulate inner haircell cilia.

9) The three type of otoacoustic emissions are: *transient evoked otoacoustic emissions (TEOAE), distortion-product otoacoustic emissions (DPOAE)*, and *spontaneous otoacoustic emissions (SOAE)*.

10) The otoacoustic emission may result from haircell motility. That is, the motion of the outer haircells in response to sound stimulation may cause additional motion of the basilar membrane, which causes the membrane to vibrate as if a sound were present and this is propagated back to the middle ear.

11) Afferent fibers: *Radial (Type I)* from inner haircells, Outer *Spiral (Type II)* from outer haircells. Efferent fibers: *Lateral olivary fibers* (LOC-crossed and uncrossed) which synapse on inner haircell axons, *Medial olivary fibers* (MOC-crossed and uncrossed) which synapse on outer haircells.

12) The *Type I fibers* carry information about sound from the inner haircells to the brainstem.

13) Axons from the apex are in the middle of the auditory nerve bundle, while those from the lower turns of the cochlea wrap around these apical fibers, so that the outside of the auditory nerve bundle contains fibers from the base of the cochlea.

14) Afferent fibers take information from the periphery up to the brainstem and central nervous system. Efferent fibers take information from the brainstem and central nervous system down to the periphery. Afferent fibers can provide both excitatory and inhibitory synaptic stimulation, whereas efferent fibers tend to be inhibitory.

15) The efferent fibers synapse on the axons of the inner haircells and directly on the outer haircells.

16) The *MOC efferent fibers* may help control the slow motility of outer haircells.

17) The stapes moves in synchrony with the vibrating source producing the sound. The stapes moves the oval window, which causes the fluids of the cochlea to vibrate in synchrony with the stapes. This vibratory pattern causes a traveling wave motion to be generated along the cochlear partition. The differential motion between the basilar and tectorial membranes caused by the traveling waves shear the cilia of the haircells. When the cilia are sheared an action potential is generated in the haircell and a neural discharge is sent long the auditory nerve. The discharges from Type I fibers connected to inner haircells carry information about sound to higher auditory centers. The shearing of the cilia of the outer haircells causes the outer haircells to be motile, which apparently helps establish an efficient coupling between the basilar and tectorial membranes, which in turn allows for the high sensitivity and frequency resolving capacity of the inner ear.

ADVANCED PROBLEMS

1) Extratympanic AP measurements are less sensitive than transtympanic measures because the measuring electrode is further away from the auditory nerve which is the source of the AP.

2) Infants are difficult to test with behavioral measures and one would not want to use invasive techniques such as putting electrodes into the middle ear. Otoacoustic measures only require a small microphone and speaker to be placed into the outer ear and are, therefore, not invasive. Finally, otoacoustic emissions do not occur if haircells and auditory nerves are not functioning correctly. Thus, a lack of an emission may indicate a problem with the function of the inner ear.

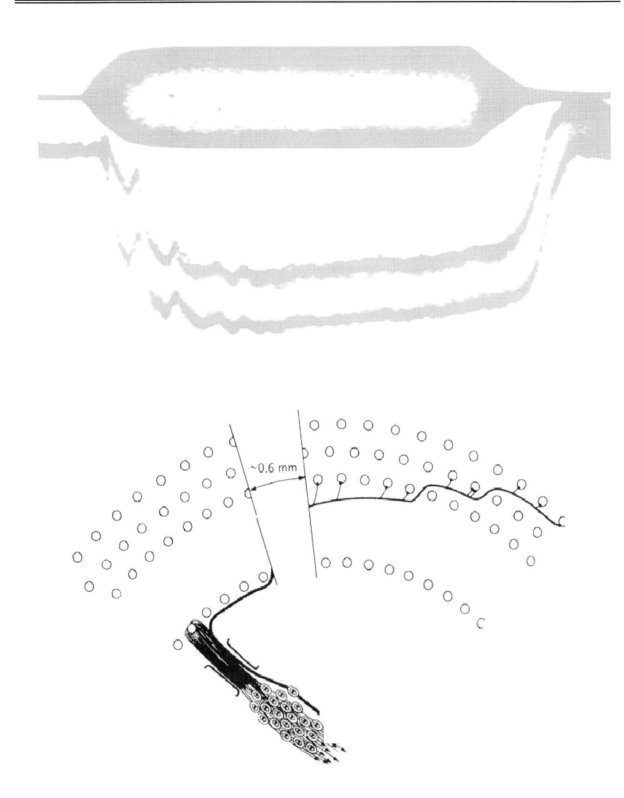

~0.6 mm

Chapter 9 - The Neural Response and the Auditory Code

CD-ROM, Web Site, ASA Tapes: The CD-ROM and Web Site (*www.parmly.luc.edu/*) should be consulted.

Instructional Hints: An analogy is often made to a gun firing a bullet as a way to explain the all-or-none law of neural transduction. It doesn't matter how hard the trigger is pulled, as long as it is pulled hard enough. The bullet leaves the gun with the same velocity independent of how hard the trigger is pulled. Thus, as long as the stimulus reaches a threshold value a spike is triggered in a similar all-or-none manner.

It is important for the student to understand that spontaneous activity is a random process. The number of neural spikes that occurs every second varies about some mean with some variance. In many experiments, the mean and variance of the spontaneous activity are measured, and then a statistical rule (such as one standard deviation above the mean) is used to define threshold.

At high levels not only does a single nerve fiber reach saturation, but the firing rate for most nerve fibers become saturated. Thus, a single fiber cannot singal a change in level. And, since there is little difference between fibers in their firing rates, there is a reduced ability to distinguish one frequency from another.

Any efferent effects will be slow acting, since it takes time for the neural singal to travel up the auditory nerve to the brainstem and then back down to the haircell and/or auditory nerve. Thus, any efferent effects, such as protection against loud sounds, would only be beneficial it there was a delay.

Both two-tone suppression and the generation of distortion products, such as the cubic difference tone, are manifestations of nonlinear processes in the cochlea. However, it is not necessarily the case that a single nonlinear process is responsible for both of these nonlinear phenomena.

The historical debate between the place and temporal theories of hearing is briefly discussed in Chapter 1, and a more detailed discussion can be found in Section 1 of the Hearing Tutorial at *www.parmly.luc.edu/*. The place code for frequency coding is like a old-fashioned switchboard. Each light on the switchboard indicates a particular phone number just like each nerve fiber in the VIIIth nerve bundle represents a different frequency.

Chapter 9 - Suggested Problems for Students

1) At the end of this chapter are several sample drawings that can be used to test students about tuning curves, response areas, input-output functions, and neural histograms of various types.

2) How does the *whole-nerve AP* differ from a single neuron action potential?

Problems 3-7: Table of the number of spikes per second recorded from one auditory nerve fiber as a function of the frequency and level of tonal stimulation.

Cell 1			Level	dB SPL				
Freq. (Hz)	10	20	30	40	50	60	70	80
250	8	9	7	11	9	10	11	15
500	7	8	6	9	11	10	15	22
750	9	11	10	9	8	15	22	28
1000	8	11	9	9	8	15	22	30
1250	10	9	8	7	10	15	26	35
1500	11	8	9	15	20	26	38	42
2000	9	15	22	35	45	47	49	48
2500	15	24	32	45	50	49	48	47
3000	9	11	15	21	28	35	46	47
3500	7	9	11	12	15	22	29	34
4000	8	7	11	12	13	12	11	15

3) Plot the *neural input-output function* for tonal stimulation at 2,000 Hz. At what level does the neuron's firing rate appear to *saturate*?

4) At 30, 50, and 70 dB SPL plot the response area for this auditory neuron.

5) Plot the *tuning curve* for this fiber if neural threshold is defined as 15 spikes/sec.

6) What is the range of *spontaneous activity* for this fiber and according to the classification used in the textbook, is this a low, middle, or high spontaneous rate fiber?

7) What is the fiber's *CF*? What is the approximate decibel difference between the tip and the low-frequency tail of the tuning curve? Is the high- or low-frequency slope of the tuning curve steeper?

Problems 8-12: A Table showing when in time a neural response was recorded for 10 (N) presentations of the same tonal stimulus. A "1" in the table means a neural spike occurred at that moment in time and a "0" means that no spike was recorded. The stimulus started at time zero (0 ms), so that -2 and -4 ms means 2 and 4 ms before the stimulus began. Thus, reading across the row at N=1, the neuron for the first presentation of the tone discharged at 4 ms before the stimulus was turned on, when the stimulus came on (0 ms), at 4 ms after the stimulus came on, etc. When the tone was presented a second time (N=2), the neuron did not fire until 2 ms after the stimulus was turned on, etc.

Time (ms)

N	-4	-2	0	2	4	6	8	10	12	14	16	18	20	22	24	26	28	30	32
1	1	0	1	0	1	0	0	0	1	0	1	0	1	0	0	0	0	0	1
2	0	0	0	1	0	1	0	1	0	1	0	0	0	1	0	1	0	1	0
3	0	0	1	0	1	0	1	0	1	0	1	0	1	0	1	0	1	0	1
4	0	0	1	0	1	0	1	0	0	0	1	0	0	0	1	0	1	0	0
5	1	0	1	0	1	0	1	0	0	0	0	0	1	0	1	0	0	0	1
6	0	0	0	1	0	1	0	1	0	1	0	1	0	1	0	0	0	1	0
7	0	0	0	1	0	1	0	1	0	0	0	1	0	0	0	1	0	1	0
8	0	0	1	1	0	1	0	0	0	0	0	0	0	1	0	1	0	0	0
9	0	0	1	1	0	1	0	0	0	1	0	1	0	1	0	0	0	1	0
10	0	1	1	1	1	0	1	0	1	0	1	0	1	0	1	0	1	0	0

8) What is the *spontaneous rate* of this fiber in spikes/sec?

9) Plot the *PST histogram*.

10) Plot the *interval histogram*.

11) What is the most likely frequency of the stimulating tone?

12) Sketch the likely *Time-locked PST histogram* for a 200-Hz sinusoid and a 20,000-Hz sinusoid.

13) Based on the following *Time-Locked PST Histogram*, what is the likely *CF* of the fiber that was stimulated with a rarefaction click? Explain.

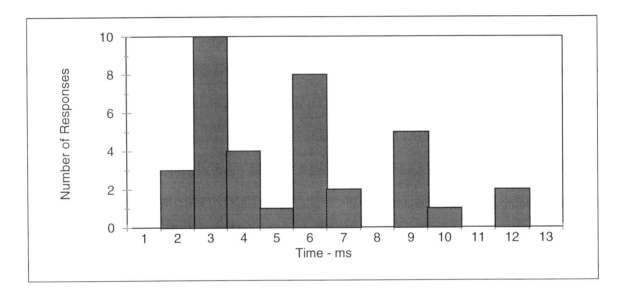

14) An auditory physiologist is measuring the neural rate of an auditory neuron in response to a sound of a particular frequency. The neuron is responding at a rate well above spontaneous activity when her graduate student accidentally turns on another stimulus and the neuron stops responding. The graduate student is bothered because he thinks that because there were no more neural responses he caused the experimenter to lose the ability to record from the neuron. What else could explain why the neuron stopped responding?

15) Describe what may happen to the neural discharge of an auditory nerve if sound is delivered to both ears as compared to when sound is delivered to only one ear.

16) Describe the two different ways in which the frequency of a tone may be encoded by the auditory nerve. What are the limitations of each "theory" (i.e., what type of tonal stimulation does each theory have trouble accounting for)?

17) Why is it unlikely that the intensity of a tone is coded by the magnitude of the neural firing rate of single auditory neurons?

18) Explain why the auditory nerve could probably not determine the temporal structure of a 10,000-Hz sound? Could the auditory nerve determine a 200-Hz amplitude modulation of a 10,000-Hz carrier tone? Explain.

19) Many sounds that we perceive in everyday life have intensities that are 60 dB or higher. What aspect of auditory neural function suggests that it is unlikely that the response rate of auditory neurons could be used to code for the important spectral aspects of sounds at these levels? What aspect of auditory nerve function might be used at higher stimulus levels?

ADVANCED PROBLEMS

1) Except for very low frequencies, do inner haircells respond to the actual displacement of the basilar membrane or to the speed (velocity) with which it moves?

2) If the Q_{10} of the low-frequency tuning curve is 1 and its bandwidth is 200 Hz, what is the CF of the tuning curve?

3) Under what conditions may the reduction of the firing rate of a neuron stimulated both ipsilaterally and contralaterally (i.e., in experiments studying the effects of the COCB) actually be due to two-tone suppression at the ipsilateral ear?

Answers for Problems for CHAPTER 9

2) The whole nerve AP is the sum of many different neural discharges from single auditory nerves, each generating its own individual action potential.

3) The neural output rate appears to saturate at around 50 dB.

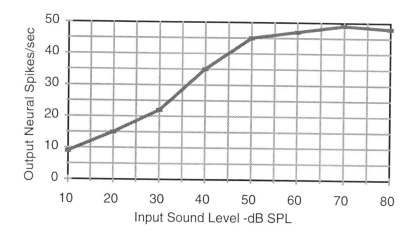

4)

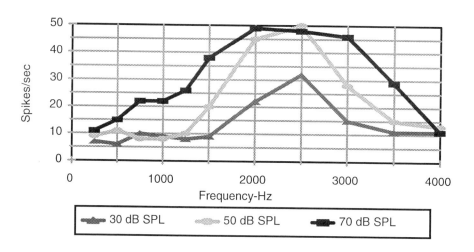

5)

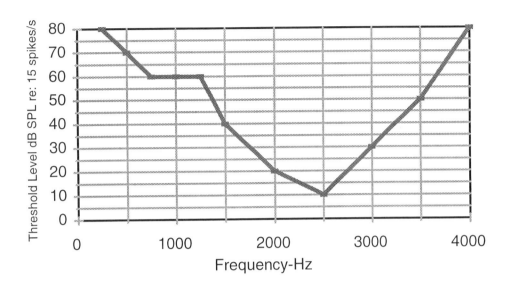

6) Since between about 6 and 11 spikes/sec there seems to be little correlation between spike rate and stimulus values, this is probably about the range of spontaneous activity for this fiber. As such this would be a medium spontaneous-rate fiber.

7) The fiber's CF is 2500 Hz, there is about 50 dB difference between CF and the low frequency tail, and the high-frequency slope of the tuning curve is much steeper than the low-frequency slope.

8) Spontaneous activity could be determined before the stimulus was turned on (at -2 and -4 ms). Out of ten presentations, the neuron fired 3 times. Thus, on average there were 0.3 spikes/ 4 ms ((3/10)*1 spike/4ms). This is 75 spikes/sec [(1,000 ms in a sec/4 ms)*0.3 spikes/sec] as an estimate of the spontaneous firing rate.

9) The PST is formed by adding up the number of spikes for each time period over the 10 presentations.

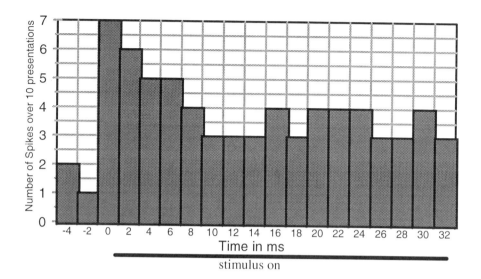

10) The Interval histogram is computed by counting the total number of intervals between successive spikes for 2, 4, 8, 12 and 16 ms between spikes.

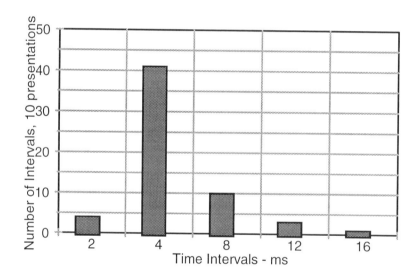

11) The stimulating tone most likely has a frequency of 250 Hz, since 4 ms and its higher integer multiples (8, 12, and 16) are the most probable intervals.

12) For 200 Hz some figure showing that 5 ms period is preserved:

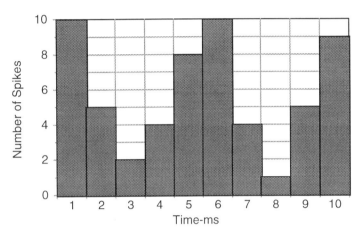

For 2,000 Hz, a flat PST since the period is too short for phase locking:

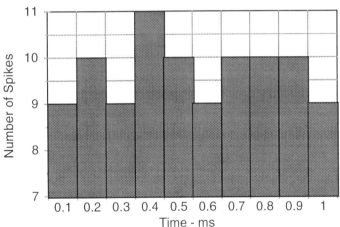

13) The best estimate of the fiber's CF is to note the times when the major peaks in the PST occur. They occur every 3 ms, suggesting that the fiber's CF is 333 Hz (1000 ms/ 3 ms).

14) It could be that the sound that was accidentally turned on was of a frequency that could inhibit the response of the fiber to the first sound. This would be an example of two-tone suppression.

15) Sound delivered to both ears could cause a lower discharge rate from a fiber recorded at one ear as compared to a case in which this fiber was recorded from when both ears were stimulated. If so, this would be an example of contralateral suppression.

16) One way for frequency to be encoded is by the place theory, which suggests that it is the nerve that discharges that carries information about frequency. Low frequencies may cause a problem for the place theory since tuning curves are broadly tuned at low frequencies and, thus, it would be difficult to tell one low-frequency sound from another. The other possible way for the auditory nerve to code for frequency is by the time between successive neural discharges, since nerve fibers discharge in synchrony with the period of stimulation. However, because of the refractory period of neural firing, such synchrony can only occur up to about 5,000 Hz.

17) Single auditory nerve fibers only change their firing rate over a 30-50 dB range and we can hear over a 140-dB range.

18) Temporal structure is probably based on fibers discharging in synchrony to the period of stimulation, but only up to frequencies of 5,000 Hz because of limitations caused by the refractory period of neural function. Thus, the temporal structure of a 10,000-Hz sound is occurring too rapidly for an auditory neuron to follow the structure. However, a 200-Hz modulation of the tone's amplitude is slow enough so that the neuron might follow this slow (5-ms period) temporal structure.

19) The firing rate of almost all auditory neurons is saturated at 60 dB SPL and tones at this high level stimulate a wide number of auditory fibers. Thus, firing rate is nearly maximal for many different fibers in the auditory nerve making it difficult for the auditory nerve to indicate any differences that might exist across frequency. The time-locked discharge rate of auditory fibers (as might be revealed by ISI histograms) still show phase-locking at 60 dB. So the auditory nerve might be able to transmit information about the frequency content of the sound by the temporal structure of the neural discharges. This is the basis of using the ALSR measure in Fig. 9.14 in the Textbook.

ADVANCED PROBLEMS

1) Inner haircells tend to respond to the velocity of basilar membrane displacement.

2) Q=CF/Bandwidth, CF=Q X Bandwidth, CF=1*200=200 Hz.

3) The appearance of contralateral suppression can really be two-tone suppression if the contralateral tone is strong enough to stimulate the ipsilateral ear. In this case, the ipsilateral ear is receiving two tones: that going directly to the ear and that which is "leaking" from the other side of the head (the contralateral ear).

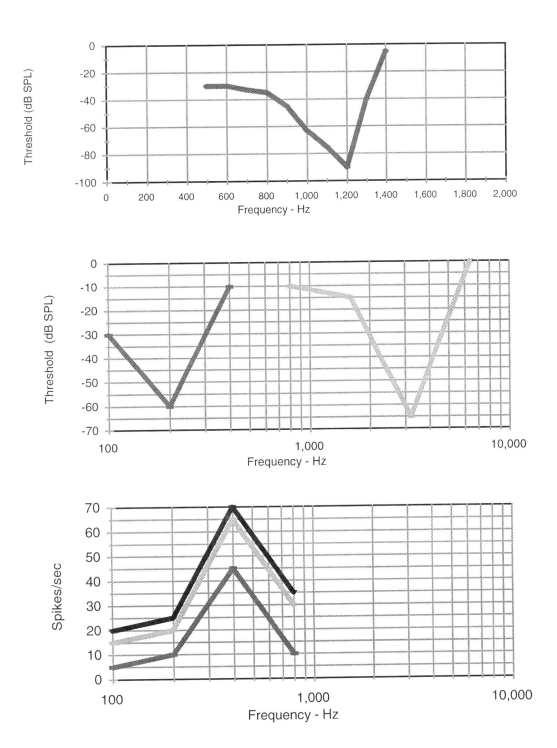

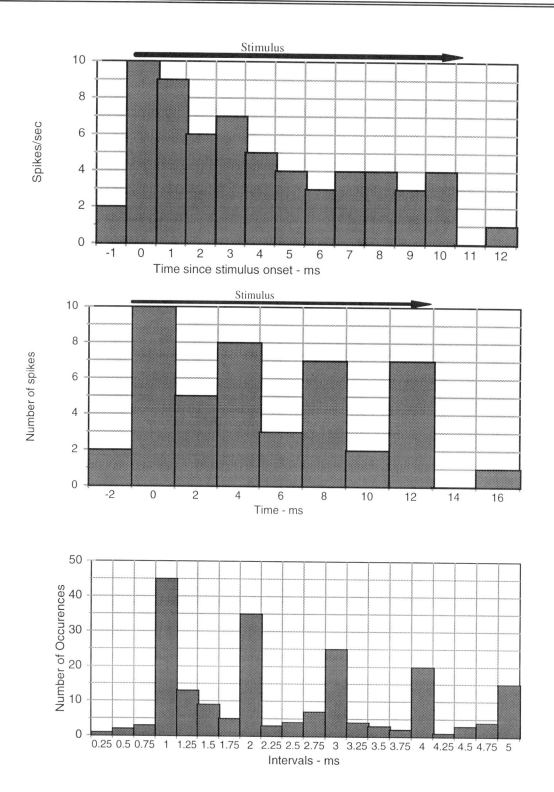

Chapter 10 - Auditory Sensitivity

CD-ROM, Web Site, ASA Tapes: The CD-ROM and Web Site (*www.parmly.luc.edu/*) should be consulted.
<u>ASA Tapes:</u> Demonstration 6, Tracks 17,18; Demonstration 8, Track 21; Demonstration 17, Track 33.

Instructional Hints: The next few chapters often require that the student be able to read graphs accurately and that they are able to replot data from one graph to another using a different format. Some students have difficulty doing this. One can accomplish two goals at the same time by having them plot psychometric functions and then find thresholds from these functions and plot the resulting thresholds. They learn about plotting and about psychophysical procedures.

Several times in this chapter, as well as in later chapters, quantities other than amplitude and intensity will be converted by taking twenty or ten times the log of a ratio. For instance, $10\log(T1/T2)$, where T1 and T2 are two temporal quantities. Such ratios are NOT decibels, but they do allow for calculations based on decibels. It might be a good idea for some students to reread Chapter 3 and Appendix A and B in the Textbook before they start Chapter 10.

While it is mentioned in the Textbook, it is worth repeating that one has to be very careful in interpreting results from discrimination experiments. When a listener is asked to tell if two sounds are different, they can base their decision on any aspect of the stimulus that allows them to make the discrimination. Often more than one stimulus attribute changes when a stimulus parameter is changed. As such, there is the possibility that the results will be confounded (see Chapter 1 in the Textbook), and it is difficult or impossible to determine which stimulus attribute led to the discrimination. Students should always be on the "lookout" for such confoundings.

Comparing data from one intensity discrimination study to another can be difficult because of the many different measures one can use. It is probably worthwhile to take a few moments to point out that one can make a soft sound (call it the masker) louder by adding a second sound (call it the signal) to it. In order to study intensity discrimination the two sounds (masker and signal) would have the same frequency. As the student should know by now, the level of the louder sound depends on the relative level of the signal and masker and on their starting phases. Thus, measures of intensity discrimination can be displayed using signal and masker levels, but only if starting phase angles are specified (as shown in Table 10.3 in Chapter 10 of the Textbook). The article by Grantham and Yost (1982) provides a table (Table II in that article) that can be used to convert from one measure of level differences to another.

Chapter 10 - Suggested Problems for Students

1) Plot the psychometric functions for the following three frequencies:

Table: Percent Correct (%) detection of tones of the given frequency and level.

Frequency (Hz)	Level in dB SPL						
	<u>10</u>	<u>12</u>	<u>14</u>	<u>16</u>	<u>18</u>	<u>20</u>	<u>22</u>
<u>500</u>	50	55	60	65	70	75	80
<u>1,000</u>	55	60	65	70	75	80	85
<u>2,000</u>	60	65	70	75	80	85	90

2) If 75% correct is used as the definition of threshold, plot the thresholds of detection as a function of the three frequencies shown in problem 1). That is, plot the three-frequency *thresholds of audibility* curve for the data shown in problem 1).

3) If 110 dB SPL was the level at which a listener experienced discomfort at 500, 1,000, and also at 2,000 Hz, what is the *dynamic range of hearing* at these frequencies given the thresholds of hearing shown in problem 1)?

4) Children in a school have their hearing tested in a sound-treated room by listening to test tones over loudspeakers. Describe and name the procedure that should be used to calibrate the listening environment so that the hearing thresholds can be compared to standardized norms.

5) After proper calibration, a student tested in the classroom described in problem 4) had thresholds of 23.9 dB SPL at 1,000 Hz, 30.6 dB SPL at 2,000 Hz, and 44.4 dB SPL at 4,000 Hz. These results suggest that the child has a hearing loss. Why? How many decibels is the hearing loss at each of the three frequencies given the Standardized Thresholds of Audibility?

6) The thresholds for hearing differ when the test tones are delivered over supra-aural headphones as opposed to insert headphones. What may cause this difference in thresholds?

7) In the laboratory, a listener's hearing is tested using headphones. The MAP calibration for that headphone at 2,000 Hz shows that with 1 volt of sound level as the input to the headphone the headphone produces 10 dB SPL as the output sound pressure level (that is, the sound pressure level in a 6-cc coupler is 10 dB SPL). The voltage into the headphone is 0.5 volts when the listener is at her threshold for detecting the 2,000-Hz tone. What is her threshold in dB SPL, given the MAP calibration data and assuming the audio equipment is operating in a linear manner. Show your calculations.

8) Your threshold for detecting a 1,000-Hz, 500-ms test tone is 10 dB SPL. Your friend's threshold for detecting a 1,000-Hz, 50-ms test tone is 20 dB SPL. In terms of sound energy, do your thresholds differ? Show your calculations.

9) The table below shows the thresholds of audibility as a function of duration for a 1,000-Hz tone. What is the best estimate of *integration time* for this listener? Explain your answer.

Threshold	**Duration (ms)**						
	10	50	100	250	500	750	1,000
(dB SPL)	30	22	20	16	14	14	14

10) The data shown in the table below are the frequency difference thresholds for discriminating a change in frequency from the standard test tone. Redo the table so that the entries are in terms of the Weber Fraction for Frequency Discrimination.

Difference Threshold	**Standard Frequency (Hz)**				
	500	1,000	2,000	4,000	8,000
(Hz)	2 Hz	4 Hz	8 Hz	16 Hz	32 Hz

11) From problem 9) what is your best guess as to the difference in frequency that this listener could discriminate if the Standard tone were 5,000 Hz? Show your calculations.

12) The Weber Fraction for Intensity Discrimination ($\Delta I/I$) for a listener is 0.25 at 1,000 Hz and 0.3 at 2,000 Hz. What are these difference thresholds in terms of ΔI in dB? Show your calculations.

13) Do the results of problem 12) represent a "near miss to the Weber fraction"? Explain.

14) The threshold for discriminating a change in the level of a noise at 20 dB SPL is about 1 dB in terms of ΔI in dB and the threshold for detecting a change in the level of a 1,000-Hz tone at 20 dB SPL is about 1.5 dB in terms of ΔI in dB. What is the difference in the Weber Fraction ($\Delta I/I$) for intensity discrimination between the noise and the 1,000-Hz tone? Show your calculations.

15) If you knew the Weber Fraction for intensity and for frequency discrimination, over approximately what range of frequencies and overall level for tonal stimuli could you predict the difference thresholds for frequency and level?

16) A student new to the study of hearing wanted to determine the ability of listeners to determine the difference in the duration of two tones as a means to study temporal discrimination. He asked listeners to discriminate between a 5- and a 10-ms tone, and in another condition between a 200- and a 400-ms tone. He found that the listeners could detect the difference between the 10- and 20-ms tones better than they could the difference between the 200- and 400-ms tones. Does this mean that

duration is the only reason that the difference thresholds are different for short-duration tones as compared to long-duration tones?

17) At a modulation rate that is less than 50 Hz, most listeners can detect that a noise is sinusoidally amplitude modulated when the depth of modulation (*m*) is about 0.05 (5%). What is this threshold in terms of 20log *m*?

18) The TMTF has the shape of a lowpass filter with a 50-Hz cutoff and a 6-dB/octave roll off (6 dB of loss in depth of modulation--20log *m*--for each octave increase in the modulation rate of the sinusoidal amplitude modulator). First, compare this lowpass filter summary with the data of Fig. 10.10 in the Textbook. This has suggested to hearing scientists that stimuli whose amplitudes change over time might be processed as if they were filtered by a lowpass filter with the description given above. If it takes -20 dB depth of modulation (i.e., 20log m = -20 dB) to just detect that a sound is modulated at 50 Hz, what must one do to the depth of modulation according to the lowpass filter described above in order to just detect the changing amplitude of a sound that is modulated at 200 Hz?

19) A communications technician has an idea that he can speed up the time to transmit a Morse Code message of short and long noise bursts (i.e., a short noise burst is a "dot" and a long noise burst is a "dash") by sending the noise bursts at a rate of 200 Hz. That is, the short (dots) and long (dash) noise bursts occur at the rate of 200 times per second. From the viewpoint of hearing, is this a good idea?

ADVANCED PROBLEMS

1) People exposed to loud sounds (e.g., those who fire guns) often have more hearing loss in the region of 4,000 Hz. Why?

2) A person's hearing is tested for bone-conduction at 2,000 Hz and it is found that the threshold for detecting a sound when the vibrator is placed on the mastoid is 48 dB re: 1 dyne. Does this person have a hearing loss? If so, how much?

3) Why might the bone-conduction hearing thresholds be lower when a vibrator is placed on the Mastoid versus the Forehead?

4) A very long tone (1-sec tone) produces a threshold of 10 dB SPL and a short tone (50 ms) produces a threshold of 20 dB; what is the value of C (the constant) in the temporal integration formula? Using the formula, what is the predicted threshold for a 150-ms tone?

5) If in an intensity discrimination experiment the more intense tone to be discriminated is generated by adding a tone (of the same frequency) to the Standard tone, then the phase at which the two tones are added is crucial for deciding what the Weber Fraction will be. Why?

6) Table 10.3 in the Textbook shows formulae for determining different measures of intensity discrimination. When two tones are added together to produce the louder tone, one tone is called the signal and the other tone (the Standard tone) is called the masker. The signal (S) to masker (M) ratio (S/M) is shown in the table to be $\{[\Delta I/I + \cos(\alpha)]^{1/2} - \cos(\alpha)\}^2$, where α is the phase angle of addition between S and M. Show that S/M equals $\Delta I/I$ when α is 90°. That is, for the case in which two tones are added together to produce the more intense tone in an intensity discrimination experiment, the Weber fraction ($\Delta I/I$) is the same as the ratio of the signal to the masker level (S/M), if the signal and masker (the two tones) are added with a 90° phase difference.

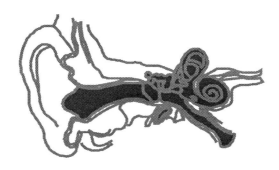

85

Answers for Problems for CHAPTER 10

1)

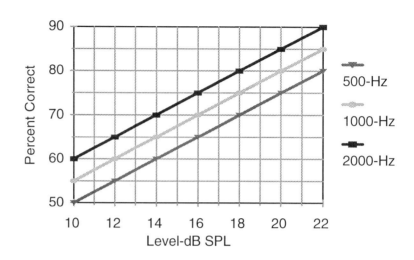

2)

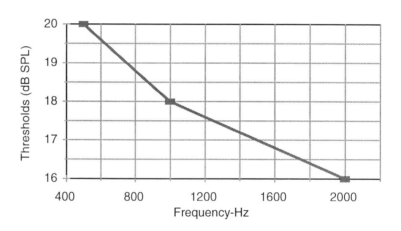

3) The dynamic range-- at 500 Hz: 110dB-20dB = 90 dB, at 1,000 Hz: 110dB-18dB = 92 dB, and at 2,000 Hz: 110dB-16dB = 94 dB.

4) A Minimum Audible Field (MAF) calibration procedure would be required. A calibrated microphone would be placed at the position of the listener's head (without the listener being present). The listener and the microphone should be approximately one meter from the loudspeaker. The sound pressure level recorded from the microphone for a given input to the loudspeaker would be determined. Then, this input level and its known sound pressure-level output would be used to determine the sound pressure level when the listener is tested using other input levels for the loudspeaker.

5) The hearing levels would all be above those in the Standard, thus indicating a hearing loss: at 1,000 Hz: 23.9dB- 2dB = 21.9 dB, at 2,000 Hz: -1.5dB-30.6dB = 32.1 dB, and at 4,000 Hz:-6.5dB-44.4dB = 50.9 dB.

6) Since insert phones are placed in the outer ear, then the outer ear resonances may not be the same as those found when sound is presented from a headphone that fits on the outside of the outer ear.

7) If a 1-volt input produces a 10-dB SPL output, a 0.5 volt input will produce half as much output, which would be an output of 4 dB SPL, i.e., $20\log(0.5/1) = 20\log(0.5) = -6$ dB; and 10-6 = 4 dB.

8) Since the tones differ by a factor of 10 in duration and in level (i.e., a 10-dB change in level is a factor of 10 in energy; $10 \log(10) = 10$ dB), the energy of the two tones is the same.

9) The best estimate of integration time is between 250 and 500 ms, since the thresholds do not change for durations longer than 500 ms.

10) For all Standard Frequencies the Weber Fraction is 0.004 or 0.4% (e.g., 2/500 = 0.004 and 32/8000 = 0.004).

11) If the Weber Fraction is 0.004 and the Standard Frequency is 5,000 Hz, then Δf is 20 Hz; $\Delta f = f$ x C, 5,000 Hz x 0.004=20 Hz.

12) To get $\Delta I/I$ from ΔI in dB recall that, $10\log(\Delta I/I+1)=\Delta I$ in dB. So, at 1,000 Hz: $10\log(1.25)=0.97$ dB, and at 2,000 Hz: $10\log(1.3)=1.14$ dB.

13) No, while the two thresholds differ, the difference is due to using different *frequencies*. The "near miss to Weber's law" refers to cases in which the Weber Fraction does not remain constant for intensity discrimination when the *level* of the sound is changed.

14) To solve this problem use the inverse of the calculations shown for problem 12). For the tone: 1 dB = $10 \log(\Delta I/I+1)$, $10^{1/10} = 1.26 =\Delta I/I+1$; $\Delta I = 1.26-1 = \mathbf{0.26}$. For the noise $10^{1.5/10} = 1.41 = \Delta I/I+1$; $\Delta I = 1.41- 1 = \mathbf{0.41}$.

15) Both Weber fractions remain relatively constant over a mid-frequency range of 400 to 4,000 Hz and a mid-level range of approximately 30 to 70 dB, except for the near miss to Weber's law for intensity discrimination.

16) Recall that the absolute threshold for detecting a 10-ms tone is lower than that for detecting a 5-ms tone, while there is little difference in the absolute thresholds for detecting a 200- or 400-ms tone. Also, recall that short-duration tones have a large spectral region over which their energy is

splattered. This makes it possible to detect energy in frequency regions that are different from that of the tonal frequency. At longer durations the energy is not spread very far from that of the tonal frequency. Thus, either differences in absolute threshold or in detecting the splatter of energy away from the frequency of the test tones may have caused the difference in duration thresholds.

17) 20log m = 20 log (0.05) = 20 X -1.3 = **-26 dB.**

18) 200 Hz is two octaves from 50 Hz, so there is a 12-dB difference in the output level of the filter, since the lowpass filter rolls off at 6 dB/octave. Thus, the input modulation depth would have to be increased by 12 dB in terms of 20log m to maintain the same level of detection. Thus, the depth of modulation would have to be -8 dB to be just detected at 200 Hz.

19) At a rate of change of 200 Hz, the TMTF shows that listeners require a lot more depth of modulation to detect temporal fluctuations in the amplitude of a sound than at lower rates. Thus, having the noise bursts presented at a 200-Hz rate may make it difficult to discern the difference between the dots (short bursts) and the dashes (long bursts).

ADVANCED PROBLEMS

1) The outer ear resonates in the region of 4,000 Hz. Thus, intense sounds (like those from gunshots) may cause even greater levels in the outer ear in the spectral region of 4,000 Hz. This increase level in the region of 4,000 Hz may be enough to cause a hearing loss.

2) The Standardized Hearing Level for a vibrator placed on the Mastoid is 31 dB re: 1 dyne at 2,000 Hz. Thus, a threshold of 48 dB represents a 17 dB hearing loss.

3) The Mastoid is closer to the inner ear than the Forehead.

4) $10\log(T(I-I_\infty))=C$, $10\log(T) + 10\log(I-I_\infty) = C$, since $(I-I_\infty)$ is already in dB as 20dB-10dB = 10 in dB. $10\log(50/1,000)+10 = -13+10 =$ **-3 = C.**

$(I-I_\infty) = 10\log(T)-C$. $(I-I_\infty) = 10\log(150/1,000)+3 = -8.2+3=5.2$ dB, so $5.2 = I-10$; I = **15.2 dB**.

5) The sum of two sinwaves of the same frequency is a function of the levels and phases of both tones. The sum is a vector sum.

6) $\{[\Delta I/I + \cos(\alpha)]^{1/2} - \cos(\alpha)\}^2$, when $\alpha=90°$ is $\{[\Delta I/I + \cos(90°)]^{1/2} - \cos(90°)\}^2$. Since $\cos(90°)$ is 0, then $\{[\Delta I/I+0]^{1/2} - 0\}^2 = \{(\Delta I/I)^{1/2}\}^2 = \Delta I/I.$

Chapter 11 - Masking

CD-ROM, Web Site, ASA Tapes: The CD-ROM and Web Site (*www.parmly.luc.edu/*) should be consulted.
<u>ASA Tapes:</u> Demonstration 2, Track 2-6; Demonstration 3, Track 7. Demonstration 9, Track 22.

Instructional Hints: Masking can take on many meanings. In the study of hearing masking should only refer to the elevation in the threshold of the signal due to the presence of the masker. If a signal is at or below its masked threshold, this does not mean that there is no information about the signal available to the nervous system. In Chapter 12 when the masking-level difference (MLD) is explained, it will be shown that a signal that is masked in one condition (e.g., the MmSm condition) can be very detectable in another condition (e.g., MoSπ) even though there is no change in the masker or signal level. There are many other such examples in the psychoacoustics literature. The student should be reminded that when a signal is added to a masker the level of the combined sound depends on the levels, starting phases, and frequencies of the signal and masker. For instance, the sum of two tones of the same frequency, level, and starting phase increases by a factor of 2 (6 dB in pressure), while the sum would increase by a factor of 1.414 (3 dB in pressure) if there was a 90° difference in the starting phases.

The concept of the critical band is very important for understanding much of the literature in hearing. The notch-noise experiment has become the accepted standard for directly measuring the critical band, although there are many other very good techniques. The notch-noise measure is preferred over using a single band of noise, because with a single band of noise listeners can attend to frequency regions above that of the signal to gain a better signal-to-noise ratio ("off-frequency listening"). Off-frequency listening leads to wider critical band estimates. As stated in the Supplement to Chapter 12 in the textbook, the critical ratio should only be used as an estimate of the critical band width when the assumption that the power in the critical band equals the power of the signal at masked threshold is true. Otherwise, the critical ratio prediction is invalid.

In many complex sound environments one is interested in detecting or processing a changing "signal" when masker(s) are present. When the signal changes in spectrum then one needs to consider the excitation pattern generated by the masker(s), in order to estimate how the signal might be processed. Moore (1986) provides many examples of using critical bands and excitation patterns.

While the schematic diagram of Figure 11.12 in the Textbook describes the general trend in masked thresholds for various temporal masking conditions, the exact nature of temporal masking varies considerably as a function of several stimulus variables. One explanation of backward masking is that the weaker signal (weaker since it is near its threshold) travels more slowly through the nervous system than does the more intense masker. Thus, the masker may reach a neural center where detection occurs before the signal does. Thus, at this neural center the signal is "simultaneously" masked. The caution about the interpretation of "suppression" expressed in the Textbook should be carefully explained to the students.

Chapter 11 - Suggested Problems for Students

1) The threshold for detecting a 1,000-Hz tone is 20 dB when no other sounds are present. When a 1,050-Hz tone is presented at the same time as the 1,000-Hz tone, the threshold for detecting the 1,000-Hz tone is 30 dB. Is there masking? If so, which tone is the signal and which is the masker? How much masking is there in decibels?

2) In the description of problem 1), is the masking task best described as; "detecting the signal" or "discriminating the signal-plus-masker presentation from the masker-alone presentation"?

3) The data shown below (psychometric functions) were collected in a psychophysical tuning-curve experiment.

Table: Percent correct in detecting a difference between a signal-plus-masker presentation and a masker presentation as a function of masker level for different masker frequencies. The signal was a 50-ms, 1,000-Hz tone presented at 10 dB SL.

Masker Frequency (Hz)	Masker Level (dB SL)							
	10	15	20	25	30	35	40	45
900	50	50	50	60	70	80	90	100
950	50	60	70	80	90	100	100	100
1,000	70	80	90	100	100	100	100	100
1,025	50	50	60	70	80	90	100	100
1,050	50	50	50	50	50	60	70	80

If 70% correct is the definition of threshold, plot the psychophysical tuning curve for these data.

4) The Table below describes a hypothetical tuning curve for a single auditory neuron. This neuron is tuned to 2,000 Hz (CF = 2,000 Hz). Recall that the neural tuning curve indicates the level of a tone required to produce a given spike rate (the threshold spike rate), such that tones with frequencies near the neuron's CF require the lowest level to elicit this threshold spike rate. Thus, if a signal of 2,000 Hz was presented at 20 dB SPL, this nerve would fire at its threshold rate. In a psychophysical tuning-curve experiment, the level of the masker must be intense enough to make it difficult to discriminate a difference between the signal-plus-masker and the masker-alone presentations. Assume that if the neuron discharges at its threshold rate when the masker alone is present, then the neuron would be firing at almost the same rate when the signal-plus-masker and the masker alone were presented. Further assume that when the nerve is discharging at about the same rate, the auditory system has difficulty discriminating between a signal-plus-masker and a masker-alone presentation (i.e., masking has occurred). For instance, if the masker were 10,000 Hz, the nerve would not

respond (except for an extremely high masker level) when the masker was presented by itself, and the nerve would fire at is threshold level when the signal-plus-masker was presented. That is, the 10,000-Hz masker does not excite this neuron and there would be essentially no masking for a 10,000-Hz masker and the 2,000-Hz signal. Given these assumptions, and the data given in the Table below, plot the predicted psychophysical tuning-curve for masker frequencies of 1,800; 1,900; 2,100 and 2,200 Hz.

Table: The level of tones of different frequencies required to elicit a threshold spike rate from this neuron.

Tonal Frequency (Hz)	Threshold Tonal Level (dB SPL)
1,750	50
1,800	45
1,850	35
1,900	30
1,950	25
2,000	20
2,050	35
2,100	50
2,150	65
2,200	80
2,250	95

5) In problem 4) it was assumed that the neural output of a single neuron tuned to the signal frequency might be the basis for describing the results from a psychophysical tuning-curve experiment, where the signal frequency is kept constant. Masking can also be measured for a fixed masker frequency and listeners are asked to detect signals of different frequencies (masking pattern experiment). In this case what is varied to determine masking? If masking is mediated by neurons tuned to the signal frequency, can detection in the masking pattern experiment be determined by a single neuron? Explain.

6) What are the three cues that a listener might use in discriminating a difference between the signal-plus-masker and the masker-alone presentation in a masking pattern experiment?

7) The machinery at a factory puts out tonal-like sounds that are different in frequency for different pieces of equipment and all of the pieces of equipment produce sounds of about the same level. It is sometimes difficult to detect if two different pieces of equipment are both on because the sounds mask each other. Even if the frequencies of the two pieces of equipment are different there can still be considerable masking. Suppose you find that one piece of equipment has a frequency of 2,000-Hz and another has frequencies in the range of 4,000 Hz and you can adjust the frequency of the higher-pitch piece of equipment over a small range near 4,000 Hz. If you want to maximize the ability to

detect that both pieces of equipment are on, why would it be best to adjust the frequency of the higher-pitch piece of equipment to be about 4,003 Hz?

8) Most hearing aids amplify the sounds that surround the listener. If one wants to detect a particular sound, what aspect of hearing means that amplifying all sounds may not help in detecting a particular sound?

9) The Table below describes the results from a band-narrowing, noise-masking experiment.

Table: Percent correct discriminations in detecting a 1,000-Hz signal in a background of noise of different bandwidths.

Masker Bandwidth (Hz)	Percent Correct
0-4,000	60
500-1,000	60
800-1,200	60
900-1,100	60
950-1,050	80
975-1,025	100
990-1,010	100

Given these data, estimate the width of the critical band?

10) Why is the critical band concept consistent with an internal filter based on a tuning curve?

11) The data below are from two different notch-noise experiments. In one experiment the signal level was 40 dB SPL and in the other experiment the signal level was 70 dB SPL. Which condition (which signal level) suggests a broader internal filter? Explain.

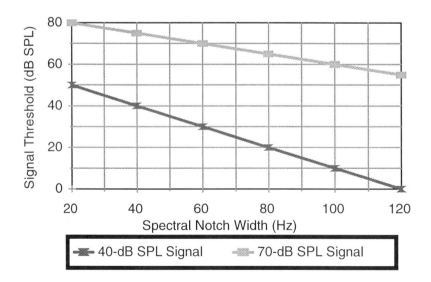

12) Given the formula for the ERB given in the Textbook what are the ERBs for filters centered at 200, 2,000, and 20,000 Hz?

13) The Table below shows the attenuation factors for internal filters for three different neurons, each tuned to a different frequency (500, 1,000, and 2,000 Hz). Suppose that in a masking pattern experiment, the masker frequency was 1,000 Hz. Plot the three-point excitation pattern for this 1,000-Hz masker.

Table: The weighting values (dB) of three Internal Filters at three different input frequencies.

Input Frequency	Internal Filter One (500-Hz CF)	Internal Filter Two (1,000-Hz CF)	Internal Filter Three (2,000-Hz CF)
500 Hz	0	-25	-40
1,000 Hz	-30	0	-20
2,000 Hz	-60	-27	0

14) What aspect of the derivation of the excitation pattern leads to the fact that low-frequency sounds appear to mask high-frequency sounds more than high-frequency sounds mask low-frequency sounds (the *upward spread of masking* effect)?

15) Most people who have a hearing loss have a high-frequency hearing loss. In designing a hearing aid, why might it not be a good idea to amplify low-frequency sounds the same as high-frequency sounds?

16) Describe how masking changes when a signal and masker are presented non-simultaneously. Be sure to use the correct terms to describe the various signal and masker temporal configurations.

17) In designing a video game, a loud sound came on before an important soft sound and as such the soft sound was often masked. To solve this problem the designer simply made the soft sound come on first before the loud sound came on. Would this actually solve the masking problem?

18) Which case describes masking results from a simultaneous-masking experiment and which case results from a forward-masking experiment. In both cases there is a 1,000-Hz signal:

Case 1: Masker Threshold Level at 1,000 Hz is 20 dB
        Masker Threshold Level at 1500 Hz is 50 dB
Case 2: Masker Threshold Level at 1,000 Hz is 10 dB
        Masker Threshold Level at 1500 Hz is 50 dB

19) In the suppression-tone experiment why is there more masking when the suppression tone is very nearly the same frequency as the masking tone?

20) For the data shown below from a suppression-tone masking experiment at which frequency is Tone B (suppressor) suppressing the masking effects of Tone A (masker). Plot the data in the same form as those plotted in Fig. 11.14 (the Suppression-Tone Experiment) in the Textbook. Signal frequency is 1,000 Hz.

Frequency (Hz) Tone A	Frequency (Hz) Tone B	Threshold Signal Level (dB)
1,000	no Tone B	50
1,000	900	55
1,000	950	60
1,000	1,000	65
1,000	1,050	45
1,000	1,100	50

ADVANCE PROBLEMS

1) If the signal is measured in units of energy (E) and the masker is measured in terms of spectrum level (No, noise power/Hz), show that the signal-to-noise ratio (E/No) is unitless. That is, the E/No ratio is not in units of time, Hz, etc.

2) Suppose a filter is triangular in shape with a base width of 500 Hz and a height of 1. Keeping the same height, what is the ERB for this filter. [Area of a triangle is 1/2(Height X Width)].

3) What is the Critical Ratio estimate of the critical bandwidth if signal power at threshold is 50 dB and the spectrum level of the masking noise is 30 dB.

4) Is the Critical Ratio a valid way to estimate the width of the critical band filter if the power of the just-detectable signal is proportional (not equal, but proportional) to the total power within the critical-band filter?

5) Plot a ROEX filter for fo=1,000 Hz, and the ERB=100 Hz. Use frequencies (f) from 500 to 2,000 Hz in 100-Hz increments.

6) Describe a situation in which the signal-to-masker ratio may be greater at a frequency that is not the signal frequency (i.e., a case where off-frequency listening might occur).

Answers for Problems for CHAPTER 11

1) Yes, there is masking since the threshold of the signal was elevated in the presence of the 1,050-Hz tone. Signal: 1,000-Hz tone; Masker: 1050-Hz tone; 10 dB of masking.

2) Since both a signal and masker are presented it is best to use signal-plus-masker and masker-alone.

3)

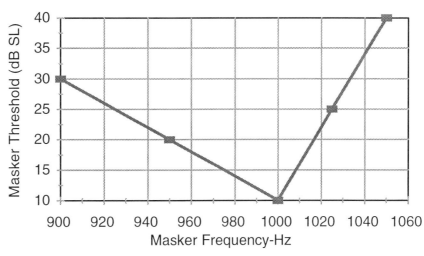

4)

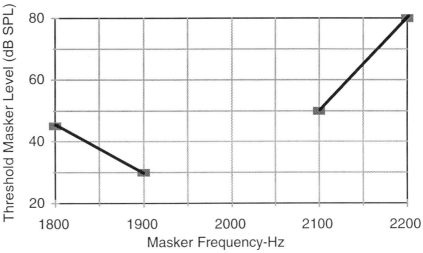

5) The level of the signal and the frequency of the signal are varied. No, there would need to be a neuron for each signal frequency. That is, the auditory system would monitor a different neuron for each signal frequency.

6) The pitch of the signal, beating caused by an interaction of aural harmonics of the masker and the signal frequency, and non-linear distortion tones caused by a non-linear interaction of the masker-plus-signal frequencies.

7) The 4,003-Hz tuning would cause this tone to beat with the aural harmonic of 4,000 Hz related to the 2,000-Hz frequency of the other piece of equipment. As such the beating could make the two pieces of equipment easier to detect than if there was no beating.

8) Amplifying all sounds will not change the signal-to-noise ratio. The signal will increase by the same amount as the masking sounds. Since signal detection is about the same as long as the signal-to-noise ratio is the same, there is no improvement caused by amplifying everything.

9) The critical bandwidth is narrower than 200 Hz (the 900- to 1100-Hz condition) and wider than 50 Hz (the 975- to 1025-Hz condition), since performance improves for bandwidths narrower than 200 Hz and there is no further improvement when the bandwidth is 50 Hz wide. Thus, 100 Hz would be a good estimate of the width of the critical band.

10) In all cases the shape of the functions are like a bandpass filter which suggests that sounds with frequencies not near the center (CF) frequency are not processed as well as those near the CF.

11) Since the masking function is shallower, the masking data for the 70-dB SPL signal probably suggests a broader internal filter than do the data for the 40-dB SPL signal. A broad internal filter will require a bigger change in notch bandwidth to produce the same change in the total power in the filter as a narrow internal filter.

12) ERB=24.74(4.37F +1);
200 Hz: ERB=24.74(4.37[.2]+1)=24.74(1.874) = **46.36 Hz**
2,000 Hz: ERB=24.74(4.37[2]+1)=24.74(9.74) = **240.96 Hz**
200 Hz: ERB=24.74(4.37[20]+1)=24.74(88.4) = **2187.02 Hz**

13)

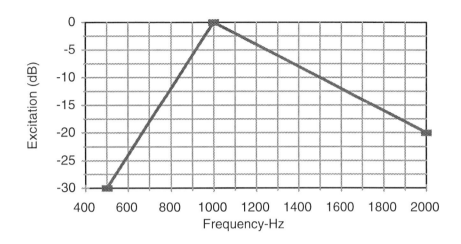

14) The tuning curves with high CFs are broader than those with low CFs.

15) If low-frequency sounds were amplified, then upward spread of masking might mask the high frequencies.

16) Most masking occurs in the forward fringe condition where the signal is at the beginning of the masker, and less masking occurs in the backward fringe condition where the signal is at the end of the masker. Then even less masking occurs in the simultaneous condition where the signal is in the middle of the masker, even less masking occurs in forward masking where the signal starts and stops after the masker is finished, and the least amount of masking occurs in backward masking where the signal starts and stops before the masker begins.

17) There could still be backward masking if the soft sound comes first, although for the same temporal separation between the signal and masker there is usually less backward than forward masking.

18) Case 2 is the forward masking condition for two reasons: There is less masking in forward masking when the signal and masker are the same frequency and the slope of the change in masking between 1,000 and 1,500 Hz is steeper in Case 2, suggesting a steeper tuning curve which occurs in forward tone-on-tone masking.

19) The suppressor tone is 20 dB more intense than the masker tone, so it can provide at least 20 dB more masking than the masker alone.

20) Since the 1,050-Hz Tone B produces less masking when it is combined with Tone A (45 dB) than when only Tone A is present (50 dB), 1,050 Hz is providing suppression.

The student needs to note that Tone A alone provides 50 dB of masking which becomes the baseline masking level (0 dB additional masking). 50 dB is subtracted from the amount of masking provided by the other Tone B.

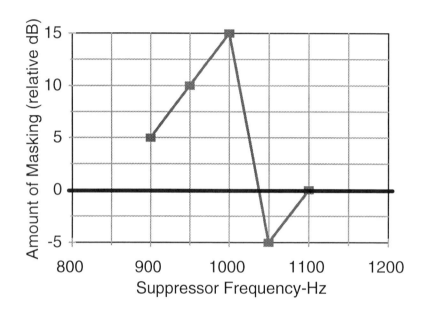

ADVANCED PROBLEMS

1) Hz has the units of 1/time, so No = power x time which has the units of energy. Thus, both the signal and the noise have units of energy, and in the ratio, these units cancel.

2) ½(500x1) = 250 = area of triangle. If unit height is assumed for the rectangle, then a width of 250 Hz would provide the same area of 250. **Thus, the ERB is 250 Hz.**

3) 50 dB - 30 dB = 20 dB = 10log(Critical Bandwidth, CBW), **so CBW is 100 Hz** (i.e., 10log(20) =100)

4) If signal threshold power is proportional to power within the internal filter then:
$Ps = k \times Pncb$, where k is a proportionality constant. Then, $CBW = Ps/(k \times No)$, and the value of k must be determined to estimate CBW.

5) Note that since ERB=4fo/p; p=4*1,000/100 = 40, with ERB=100, and fo=1,000.

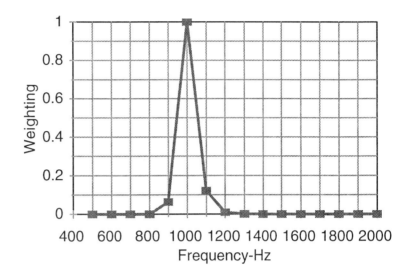

6) Any case in which the spread of excitation is such that there is less masker or more signal level in a different frequency region than that of the signal. For instance, consider a low-pass noise with a cutoff frequency of 900 Hz used to mask a 1,000-Hz signal. There will be masking noise at 1,000 Hz since the filter will roll off from 900 Hz. The excitation of activity from the 1,000-Hz signal will spread to frequencies above 1,000 Hz. Thus, there might be a greater signal-to-masker level ratio above 1,000 Hz than at 1,000 Hz, depending on how the filter function rolls off and the assumptions about the amount of the spread of excitation.

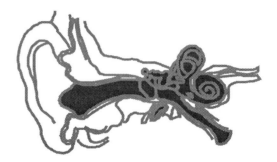

Chapter 12 - Sound Localization and Binaural Hearing

CD-ROM, Web Site, ASA Tapes: The CD-ROM and Web Site (*www.parmly.luc.edu/*) should be consulted.
<u>ASA Tapes:</u> Demonstration 37, Tracks 72-74; Demonstration 38, Tracks 75-79.

Instructional Hints: It is surprising how many people are not aware of their ability to locate objects based on the sound they produce or, if they are, they do not realize that sound has no spatial attributes. Having people close their eyes and point to where you are as you move around the room talking can reveal how well one can localize the sources of sound. It is also worth pointing out that while vision may appear to be a better sense for determining the location of objects, one cannot see behind them, but they can localize sound sources that are in the back.

Scientists and philosophers had significant difficulty accounting for sound localization since sound does not have spatial parameters. We now readily accept the idea that the attributes of sound (e.g., interaural level and time differences) can be processed by the auditory system to locate sound sources. Sound localization is a computed ability, in that the auditory periphery does not code for sound source location, but rather for the frequency, time, and level of the complex sound field. Thus, the neural cues for sound localization must be "computed" from the information contained in the peripheral code.

The use of the spectrum of sound that results from the HRTF as a cue for sound localization in the vertical plane may require some additional explanation. If the cue for vertical localization is a loss or gain of energy in some frequency region, such a spectral valley or peak could be a characteristic of the spectrum of the originating sound. Thus, how does the nervous system determine if a particular spectral feature is due to the transformation of sound caused by the HRTF or is a characteristic of the originating sound? It has been suggested that the spectral peaks and valleys caused by the HRTF may be so unusual that they rarely occur in the spectrum of natural sounds. It is also possible that comparisons of spectral peaks and valleys between the ears or over time as the head moves could help the auditory system differentiate HRTF-spectral features from those occurring for the originating sound.

The precedence effect is probably an important evolutionary feature of auditory processing. It is likely the species that could differentiate the sound coming from a source from one coming from a reflective surface would survive over a species that could not. Echoes are perceived when precedence breaks down. Recently (Litovsky et al, J. Acoust. Soc. Am. 106, 1633-1654,1999) the precedence effect is seen as a more complicated phenomenon than previously thought.

The masking-level difference (MLD) refers to detecting a signal in the presence of a masker and involves the difference between two different masking conditions. Thus, an MLD might be due to a change in one or both of the conditions. That is, a MLD for say some condition like that between MoSo and MoSπ might be due to changes in detection in the MoSo, MoSπ, or both conditions.

Chapter 12-Suggested Problems for Students

1) What are the three spatial planes and can a source be located in these three planes based only on the sound produced by the source?

2) What is the *interaural time difference* for a 500-Hz tone, if the *interaural phase difference* is 45°?

3) In the real world for real sound sources that travel directly from the source to the two ears, can the sound arrive at the left ear first and also be softer at the left ear relative to that arriving at the right ear? Explain your answer.

4) If the time it takes for sound to travel from one ear to the other ear is 800 μsec, at what frequency would this 800-μsec *interaural time difference* at stimulus onset produce a 0° *interaural phase difference* during the ongoing portion of the sinusoid? That is, there is an *interaural time difference* that is greater than zero that will lead to all peaks in the sinewave except the first peak to be in phase (see Figure 12.7 in the Textbook).

5) Suppose the following data were obtained for two different sound sources:

	Sound Source A	Sound Source B
Interaural level difference	8 dB	-8 dB
(left ear - right ear)		

Where are the two sound sources in relation to each other and to midline (midline means directly in front of the listener)?

6) According to the *Duplex Theory of Localization*, why is it more difficult to accurately localize sound sources with frequencies in the region of 1,500 Hz than in lower or higher frequency regions?

7) Describe how an *MAA* (minimal audible angle) threshold is obtained.

8) How does the *MAA* change with frequency and with the position of the standard sound?

9) Suppose that the smallest *interaural time difference* an animal can discriminate is 100 μsec and that the speed of sound is approximately 14 inches/ms. If an animal's head is too small in diameter, the time it takes sound to travel from one ear to the other will be less than 100 μsec. What is the

approximate head size diameter at which the *interaural time difference* would be less than 100 μsec (that is, animals with heads smaller than this diameter could not localize on the basis of *interaural time differences*).

10) The bones and other structures of the fish head are about the same impedance as water. Thus, sound travels through a fishe's head about the same as does through the surrounding water. Why would this make it difficult for *interaural level differences* to be a useable cue for localization for fish?

11) You are sitting in your apartment and you hear a car engine "backfire." You are almost certain that the backfire-sound came from the direction of the building next to yours and not from the street. This doesn't seem possible, since a car could not be in the building. You figure that what you heard was the echo of the backfire-sound from the wall of the building. If so, what "law" of hearing was "broken" and why?

12) From the diagram below, which sound locations (A, B, C, and D) might be confused with each other, if the listener does not move their head and only interaural differences are used for sound localization?

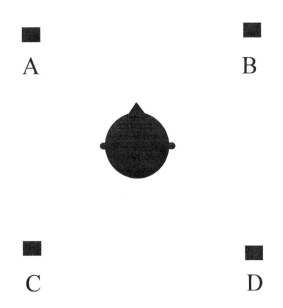

13) How might the existence of the *pinna* make the localization confusions described in Problem 12) less confusing?

14) If the *HRTF* is useful for localizing sounds in the vertical direction, why would the *HRTF* cues be more useful for high-frequency sounds than for low-frequency sounds? (Hint: consider the shape of the *HRTF* amplitude spectra shown in Chapter 6 in the Textbook)

15) What are the cues for locating sound in each of the three spatial planes?

16) What is the difference between *sound localization* and *lateralization*?

17) Listeners can detect a small change in the *interaural level difference* of a low-frequency tone in a *lateralization* task, but according to the *Duplex Theory of Localization* they cannot localize a low-frequency tone in a real acoustic environment on the basis of interaural level. Why are these two observations not inconsistent?

18) Can listeners discriminate *interaural time differences* and *interaural level differences* at 250 Hz? At 500 Hz? At 1,000 Hz? At 3,500 Hz? Explain

19) What is the full statement of the *Duplex Theory of Sound Localization?*

20) Would the *interaural time difference* threshold be about the same or very different for a single transient (impulse) signal that is high-passed filtered at 4,000 Hz as compared to that for a train of transient signals repeated at 300 times per second and then high-pass filtered at 4,000 Hz?

21) If one wants to recreate a good sense of real-world spatial location when complex stimuli are presented over headphones, what else in addition to providing proper *interaural time and level differences* needs to be provided in the playback system?

22) A person is listening to a noise-masked tonal signal when the noise and signal are presented to just the right headphone. What would happen to the masked threshold for detecting that tonal signal if a noise of the same frequency content, level, duration, and no interaural differences was also presented over the other headphone (i.e., left headphone)? Next, what would happen to the masked threshold of the tone when the noise is presented to both ears, and the tonal signal was also presented to the left headphone with the same frequency, starting phase, level, and duration as it was presented to the right headphone?

23) Provide the *MLD* abbreviations for the following conditions:

Masker	Signal
interaurally in phase	interaurally in phase
interaurally out of phase	interaurally in phase

presented to both ears presented to only one ear

24) The ability of the auditory system to determine interaural differences of time and level allows us to perform two types of tasks. What are these two tasks?

ADVANCE PROBLEMS

1) If a sound is turned on at one loudspeaker and then 100 ms later it is turned on at another loudspeaker which is located 45° from the first loudspeaker, what is the velocity of simulated movement of the sound?

2) If a 4,000-Hz tone is presented to one ear and a 4,003-Hz tone to the other ear, what might a listener perceive? How is this condition different and how might the perception be different from the condition in which these two tone are added together and presented to only one ear?

3) According to the *Equalization Cancellation* model (EC), which condition would produce the largest *MLD* and why: MoSm or MoS$_{II}$?

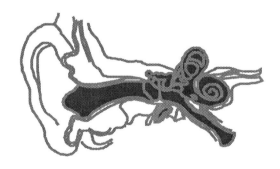

Answers for Problems for CHAPTER 12

1) The three planes are: azimuth (horizontal or left-right) plane, vertical (up-down) plane, and distance (range or near-far) plane. Yes, a sound can be located in space based on only the sound produced by the source.

2) Period of 500 Hz is 2 ms. $45°$ is 1/8 of a period ($45°/360° = 1/8$). Thus, 1/8 of 2 ms = 0.25 ms or 250 μsec.

3) In almost all cases the ear that receives the sound first also receives the louder sound, so the answer is no.

4) If the period is 800 μsec, then the frequency is 1,250 Hz (1,000,000/800). If a 1,250-Hz tone is delayed 800 μsec at one ear relative to the other ear, then the ongoing portion of the waveforms at each ear will be in phase. Thus, a 1,250-Hz tone would produce an ambiguous set of *interaural time differences*: 800 μsec time difference at the beginning of the waveform and no time differences after that (see Fig. 12.8 in the Textbook).

5) The two sources are likely to be at equal distances from midline, Source B toward the right and Source A toward the left.

6) Sounds with lower frequencies are localized on the basis of *interaural time differences* and sounds with higher frequencies are localized on the basis of *interaural level differences*. At 1,500 Hz neither interaural difference provides a very good cue for sound localization.

7) The *MAA* is obtained by determining the minimal difference in the location of two sound sources that a listener can detect.

8) The *MAA* is low at low and high frequencies (i.e., the *MAA* is high in the region of 1,500 Hz). The *MAA* is lowest when the standard is at midline (in front) and increases as the standard is moved from in front to one side.

9) 100 μsec is 1/10th of 1 ms (100/1,000). Thus, the head size would be approximately 1/10 of 14 inches or 1.4 inches. Thus, animals with head diameters of 1.4 inches or less could probably not use *interaural time differences* to locate sound sources.

10) Since the sound would travel through the head with little impedance, the head could not provide a sound shadow. As such the level at the ear opposite a sound source would be almost equal to that at the ear facing the sound source. Hence, there would be no *interaural level difference* available for sound localization.

11) The "*law of the first wavefront*" or the "*precedence effect*" would not be operating under these conditions. The precedence effect states that the sound from the source reaches the listener first (before any reflection) and as such determines the spatial location of the perceived source. In this case the location of the echo determined the perceive location of the sound.

12) A and C produce the same *interaural time and level differences*, and so do B and D. Thus A and C are on one cone of confusion and B and D on another cone of confusion.

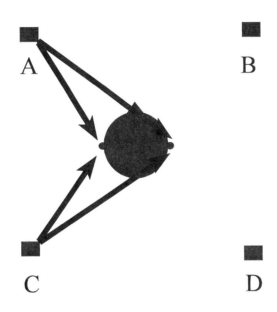

13) The *pinna* might block the sound from behind (C and D) more than that from in front (A and B), thus making it possible to differentiate between A and C and between B and D. That is, the *HRTF* for positions C and D might be different than those for A and B due to the pinna.

14) There is very little change in the amplitude or phase spectra of the *HRTF* at low frequencies. All of the changes that occur as a function of frequency appear above approximately 3,000 Hz.

15) Azimuth plane: interaural differences of time and level; vertical plane: *HRTF*, distance: loudness and early reflections.

16) *Sound localization* refers to locating real sound sources in real acoustic environments. *Lateralization* refers to determining the location of lateralized images when sound is presented over headphones.

17) While a 1-dB to 2-dB *interaural level difference* can be discriminated at low frequencies in a *lateralization* task, the actual level difference measured for real sound sources around a real head may not be that large at low frequencies. Thus, while the auditory system can detect an *interaural level difference* at low frequencies, these *interaural level differences* may not be large enough to be detected in a *sound localization* task.

18) Listeners can detect *interaural time differences* at 250, 500 and 1,000 Hz, but not at 3,500 Hz according to the data on discrimination of *interaural time differences* as a function of frequency.

19) Sounds with low-spectral frequencies or slow-temporal modulations (even if the sounds have high-spectral frequencies) can be localized on the basis of *interaural time differences*. Sounds with high frequencies can be localized on the basis of *interaural level differences*.

20) According to the modified *Duplex Theory of Sound Localization,* a single transient that is high-pass filtered is high frequency and has no temporal modulation. Thus, it would be difficult to process on the basis of *interaural time differences*. If this transient is repeated at a low rate, such as 300 times per second, then this slow temporal modulation might make it possible to process the sound on the basis of *interaural time differences*.

21) The *HRTF* for the sound at each ear would also have to be provided for the headphone delivered sound to be perceived as if it were an actual sound source in a real acoustic environment.

22) The first case is the *MmSm* case. If the noise is now added to the other ear, the condition becomes *MoSm*. In this case, there is a 10-dB *MLD* which means the masked threshold is lower. That is, adding more noise (but to the other ear) makes it easier to detect the tone. Now, if the tone is also presented to the other ear the condition becomes *MoSo*, and the threshold drops back to the *MmSm* threshold. So, adding the tone to the other ear makes it harder to detect the tone as compared to the case in which the tone is at one ear and the noise is at both ears (*MoSm*).

23)

Masker	Signal	MLD Condition
interaurally in phase	interaurally in phase	**MoSo**
interaurally out of phase	interaurally in phase	**MπSo**
presented to both ears	presented to only one ear	**MoSm**

24) The ability to process *interaural time and level differences* makes it possible for the auditory system to localize sound sources in the azimuth plane and to more easily detect signals in background maskers (i.e., an example of the "*cocktail party effect*").

ADVANCED PROBLEMS

1) The velocity of the perceived motion would be 45°/100 ms or 0.45°/ms or 450°/sec.

2) The listener might detect a "binaural beat" of 3 Hz. That is, the lateralized image might oscillate left and right in the head at a rate of 3 times per second. When the these two tones are mixed and presented to one ear, the listener would not hear any change in the position of a lateral image, but would probably perceive a change in loudness at the rate of 3 Hz (beats, see Chapters 4 and 13 in the Textbook).

3) According to *the EC* model, in the MoS_{II} condition the maskers are canceled and the signals are added. In the *MoSm* condition, the maskers are also canceled, but the signal is not doubled; it remains at its original level. Thus, in the MoS_{II} condition the signal is twice as intense as it is in the *MoSm* condition. Thus, the signal should be easier to detect in the MoS_{II} than in the *MoSm* condition. In fact, since doubling the signal intensity means a 3-dB increase, one could predict that the difference in the *MLD* between the MoS_{II} and *MoSo* conditions should be about 3 dB. The actual difference is about 5 dB (see Table 12.2 in the Textbook) which is close to the predicted value.

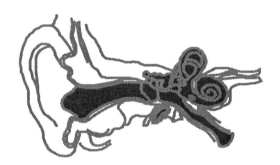

Chapter 13 - Loudness and Pitch

CD-ROM, Web Site, ASA Tapes: The CD-ROM and Web Site (*www.parmly.luc.edu/*) should be consulted.

<u>ASA Tapes:</u> Demonstration 7, Tracks 19-20; Demonstration 21, Tracks 38-39: Demonstration 25, Track 48; Demonstration 32, Tracks 62-63, Demonstration 33, Tracks 64-67, Demonstration 34, Tracks 68-69.

Instructional Hints: It is important for students to understand some of the differences between objective psychophysical measures like a *just noticeable difference (jnd)* and subjective measures like *loudness* and *pitch*. In a discrimination task a listener can be told that he or she is incorrect if two tones do not differ. However, in a task like a loudness-matching or a pitch-matching task, the listener cannot be told that they are correct or incorrect. Their judgments may not be reliable from measurement to measurement or they may not agree with other listener's judgment, but there is no absolute standard by which their *loudness* or *pitch* judgments can be correct or incorrect. Thus, measures like a *jnd* are *objective* in that the judgements that lead to the measure can be correct or incorrect. Measures like *loudness* and *pitch* are *subjective* because the judgments cannot be judged correct or incorrect.

As problem 2 suggests, a procedure like the equal-loudness procedure can be used to measure other subjective attributes of sound using a matching procedure. Annoyance is a common example. Density and volume (which are briefly mentioned at the end of Chapter 13 in the Textbook) are two other examples. The level control on a radio or stereo system may be labeled *loudness* or *volume*. Now a days these two terms are used interchangeably to indicate a control that varies sound level. Many years ago the two terms were different in that the way in which level was varied was different for *loudness* than it was for *volume*. At that time *equal-loudness contour* data were used to help design a *loudness* control and similar *equal-volume contours* were used to help design a *volume* control. In any case it is important that the level control be based on something like loudness rather than physical level. That is, when one moves the control from 2 to 4, one wants loudness not just level to vary by a factor of 2.

Any music student will find the discussion of *scales of pitch* in Chapter 13 in the Textbook to be very limited. The major point of this discussion is to provide the definition of a few terms (e.g., *semitone*) and to indicate that the musical scale is an important method for measuring *pitch*. In many experiments the pitch of a comparison sound is based on matches to sinusoids of different frequencies. Other investigators use pulse trains of different pulse frequencies because the *timbre* of the pulse train is often more similar to that of the comparison stimulus than the *timbre* of a sinusoid. Note the definition of *timbre* is one of exclusion (i.e., it is not loudness, pitch, or duration). Inclusionary definitions of *timbre* have been difficult to achieve.

Chapter 13- Suggested Problems for Students

1) Why are measures such as "*loudness*" and "*pitch*" considered "subjective"?

2) Using the equal loudness procedure as a guide and using one of the same "standard" stimuli that is used to measure loudness (i.e., a 1,000-Hz tone at 40 dB SPL), describe a procedure for determining the "annoyance" of tones of other frequencies and levels.

3) Why is each curve on the plot of equal loudness contours (Fig. 13.1 in the Textbook) called an "*equal loudness*" contour?

4) A 60-phon tone is said to be 20 dB *louder* than a 40-phon tone. Does this mean that these two tones also differ in physical level by 20 dB? Explain.

5) How does a *sone* differ from a *phon*?

6) Provide an example of why loudness does not just vary with stimulus level.

7) For the data shown below from a pitch-matching experiment, a listener adjusted the frequency of a tone so that she felt it was matched in pitch to a complex noise-like standard stimulus. What is your best guess as to the pitch (expressed in Hz) of the noise-like standard stimulus? Explain.

TRIAL	FREQUENCY IN Hz OF MATCHING TONE
1	98
2	100
3	102
4	99
5	100
6	100
7	97
8	101
9	100
10	100

8) By dividing a pitch scale, such as the *Equal Temperament Scale*, into twelve equal logarithmic intervals means that the ratio of successive frequencies in the scale is a constant. The pitch scale shown in Table 13.1 of the Textbook provides entries for the "white" notes on a piano keyboard. That is, the sharps and flats (the "black keys") are not included. A complete 12-note pitch scale might be:

C, C♯, D, D♯, E, F, F♯, G, G♯, A, A♯, B.

The "♯" means "sharp," so "C♯" is "C sharp." For the *Equal Temperament Scale* shown in Table 13.1 in the Textbook, provide the frequencies for each of these 12 notes. That is, in addition to the frequencies shown in Table 13.1 in the Textbook, provide the frequencies for the notes with sharps. (Hint: the ratio of the frequency for E to the frequency for F would be the same as that for C to C♯).

9) For each stimulus shown on the last page what might its pitch (in Hz) be (but, see Problems 10-11 before you answer this question)?

10) For one of the stimuli shown in Problem 9, it would be difficult to determine what the pitch might be. Which one is this? What is the pitch of this type of stimulus called? Although the pitch of this stimulus is not that of the fundamental (or the missing fundamental), what is the fundamental frequency for this stimulus?

11) There has been a debate for many years about the auditory mechanisms that are responsible for determining pitch. The two major proposed mechanisms are the place code for frequency coding and the temporal code based on neural units that phase lock to periodic signals. Give an example of a stimulus whose pitch would be consistent with the place theory and a stimulus whose pitch would be consistent with the temporal theory.

12) Describe how you would use the *"cancellation method"* to measure the cubic-difference tone when $f1$=600 Hz and $f2$=1,000 Hz?

13) In using the cancellation method, a listener indicated that a tone with a level of 45 dB SPL and a phase of 72° canceled the pitch of the cubic-difference tone generated when $f1$=700 Hz and $f2$=1,200. What is the best estimate of the frequency, level, and phase of this cubic-difference tone?

14) In Chapter 11, tonal masking experiments were described in which the threshold of a signal tone at different frequencies was determined when a tone at one frequency served as a masker (experiments designed to measure *excitation patterns*). For example, a 1,200-Hz signal may be presented with a 2,000-Hz masker. In this case, listeners are asked to determine if the 2,000-Hz signal plus the 1,200-Hz masker were presented or if just the 1,200-Hz masker was presented.

When the signal has a frequency that is somewhat higher than that of the masker (as in the example just given), the threshold level of the signal is near the level of the masker. Under these circumstances, the listener could determine that the signal (at 2,000 Hz) and masker (at 1,200 Hz) were presented because the level of the signal is high enough for it to be detected in the presence of the masker. It is also possible that even if the listener cannot detect the signal, they could detect the presence of a nonlinear combination tone, and as such, the detection of this combination would allow the listener to detect that the 1,200-Hz masker was not the stimulus that was presented. In this case, the listener could detect a difference between the signal-plus-masker and the masker, by detecting the presence of the combination tone and not by detecting the signal per se. The detection of the combination tone can only occur if its frequency is lower than that of the masker and the signal. For the 1,200-Hz masker and 2,000-Hz signal, which combination tones might be detectable and what are their frequencies?

15) What term is used to describe the difference between two sounds that are perceived as different but are judged to have the same frequency, the same duration, and the same level?

ADVANCED PROBLEMS

1) The pitch of the missing fundamental could be due to aspects of nonlinear distortion. How could these pitches be based on nonlinearities and what is some evidence against nonlinearities being responsible for the pitch of the missing fundamental?

2) Even though most nonlinear processes produce summation tones, they are rarely audible. Why?

3) If the "beating" procedure was used to measure the cubic-difference tone for primaries of $f1=750$ Hz and $f2=1,000$ Hz, describe the frequency of the stimuli that would be presented to the listener with the assumption that the listener would be presented a 3-Hz beating stimulus to cancel.

4) In Appendix A, the nonlinear equation $y=x+x^2$, when $x =A\sin(2\pi f1t) + A\sin(2\pi f2t)$, produced nonlinear combination tones up to $f1$-$f2$ and $f1$+$f2$. If the cube term, x^3, is added, then cubic-difference tones can be produced as well. Using the definition of x given above, the logic employed in Appendix A, and the two relationships shown below, derive the output for $y=x^3$:
$\sin^3 a = 1/4[3\sin a - \sin 3a]$, and $\sin a \sin^2 b = 1/4[2\cos a - \cos (a+2b) - \cos (a-2b)]$

A

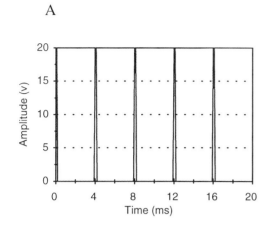

B

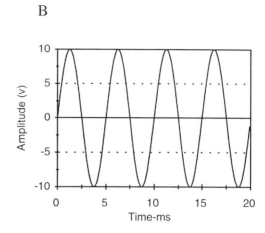

C

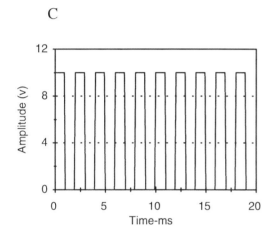

D

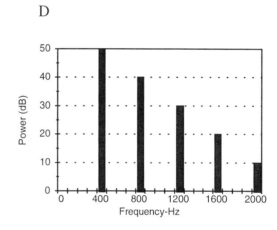

E

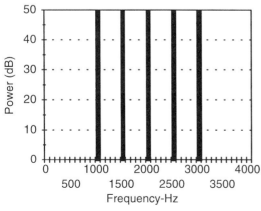

F

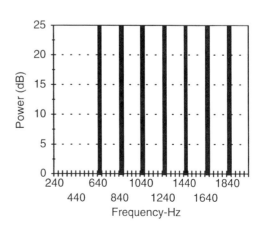

Answers for Problems for CHAPTER 12

1) *Loudness* and *pitch* are considered subjective because they are not direct correlates of a single aspect of the physical stimulus. They are judgments of the attributes of sound that cannot be judge "wrong."

2) The listener would be presented the standard stimulus and then a comparison tone at a particular frequency. The listener would adjust the level of this comparison tone until he or she felt that it was equal in "annoyance" to that of the standard. This procedure would be repeated for other frequencies of the comparison. The resulting levels would constitute an "equal annoyance contour."

3) Each equal-loudness contour indicates that all tones presented at the frequencies and levels indicated by the contour will sound equal in perceived loudness.

4) No, not at all. Note, for instance, from Fig. 13.1 in the Textbook, that a 40-phon tone at 100 Hz has a level of about 60 dB SPL, and a 60-phon tone at 1,000 Hz also has a level of about 60 dB SPL. Thus, even though the tones differ in loudness by 20 phons, they have the same physical level.

5) While *phons* and *sones* are both measures of loudness, they differ in the way they are obtained. It is the case that a 1-sone sound is a 40-phon sound.

6) Many changes in a stimulus cause a change in loudness. Under many conditions changes in duration, frequency, and bandwidth all lead to changes in perceived loudness.

7) The data from this pitch-matching experiment are as follows:

Frequency of Matching Tone	Number of Matches
97 Hz	1
98 Hz	1
99 Hz	1
100 Hz	5
101 Hz	1
102 Hz	1

Since 100 Hz was the most frequent match, the best estimate of the pitch of the noise-like standard would be 100 Hz.

8) The ratio for the *Equal-Temperament Scale* is 1.058 (e.g., 353 Hz/332 Hz). Thus, the frequencies (rounded to the nearest Hz) for all 12 notes are:

C	C♯	D	D♯	E	F	F♯	G	G♯	A	A♯	B
264 Hz	280 Hz	296 Hz	314 Hz	333 Hz	352 Hz	373 Hz	395 Hz	419 Hz	443 Hz	470 Hz	498 Hz

9) Figure A: 250-Hz pitch since the periodicity of the pulses is 4 ms; Figure B: 200-Hz pitch since this is a sinwave with a 5-ms period; Figure C: 500-Hz pitch, since this is a square wave with a 2-ms period; Figure D: 400-Hz pitch, since the fundamental frequency is 400 Hz; Figure E: 500-Hz pitch, since the missing fundamental is 500 Hz; Figure F: difficult to determine, see problem 10).

10) In Figure F it appears as if the stimulus has frequency components at 640, 840, 1,040, 1,240, 1,440, 1,640, and 1,840 Hz. That is, 200-Hz spacing, but with each frequency component shifted up 40 Hz from a stimulus with a fundamental of 200 Hz. This pitch is called the *"pitch-shift of the residue"* and its pitch would be slightly higher than 200 Hz. 40 Hz is the fundamental frequency of this waveform.

11) A sinwave or any other stimulus that has significant energy at the frequency of the reported pitch could be accounted for by a pitch theory based on the place code. The *pitch of missing fundamental* stimulus (with all tones added together in sin phase) or that of any other stimulus that does not have energy at the reported pitch but does have a temporal periodicity that repeats with an interval equal to the reciprocal of the reported pitch could be accounted for by a temporal code.

12) The cubic-difference tone in this case is 200 Hz (2*600 Hz -1,000 Hz = 200 Hz). Thus, the experimenter presents the two primaries of 600 Hz and 1,000 Hz and a *cancellation tone* of 200 Hz. The listener adjusts both the level and the starting phase of the 200-Hz cancellation tone so that he or she no longer detects a 200-Hz pitch associated with the cubic-difference tone.

13) The cubic-difference tone frequency is 200 Hz (2*700 Hz - 1200 Hz), the estimated level of the cubic-difference tone is 45 dB SPL (level is relative to the level of the primaries), and the estimated phase of the cubic-difference tone is either 252° (180° + 72°) or -108° (72° - 180°). Further note that 252° and -108° are the same phase in that 360°-108°=252° (remember that phases lie along a 360° circle).

14) Chapter 13 in the Textbook indicates that the primary difference tones (*f1-f2*) and the cubic-difference tones are audible combination tones if their frequencies are less that those of the primaries, which in this case are the masker and signal (i.e., 1,200 and 2,000 Hz). Thus, frequencies in the region of 800 Hz (2,000 Hz - 1,200 Hz = 800-Hz difference tone) and 400 Hz (2*1,200 Hz - 2,000 Hz = 400-Hz cubic-difference tone) could be detected and, therefore, could be the basis for discriminating a difference between the signal-plus-masker and the masker.

16) *Timbre* is the term used to describe the perceptual difference among sounds that have the same duration, pitch, and loudness but are distinguishable.

ADVANCE PROBLEMS

1) A stimulus which produces a missing fundamental pitch (e.g., 700, 800, 900, 1,000 Hz) can also produce a 100-Hz difference tone (e.g., 800 Hz - 700 Hz = 100 Hz). Perhaps the 100-Hz *missing fundamental pitch* is nothing more than the 100-Hz difference tone. However, noise can mask the detection of a difference tone. When a noise is presented along with the missing fundamental stimulus such that the difference tone would be masked, listeners still report that the pitch is 100 Hz, suggesting that the basis for the 100-Hz pitch cannot be the difference tone.

2) Summation tones would have frequencies that are above those of the primaries. Since low frequencies mask high frequencies very well (*upper spread of masking*), the summation tones are usually masked by the primary tones.

3) In this case the cubic-difference tone is 500 Hz (2*750 Hz - 1,000 Hz = 500 Hz). A 503-Hz (or 497 Hz) tone would beat at 3 Hz with the 500-Hz cubic difference tone. Thus, the experimenter would present the 750-Hz and 1000-Hz primaries, a 500-Hz cancellation tone, and a 503(497)-Hz beating tone.

4) $x = A\sin(2\pi f1t) + A\sin(2\pi f2t)$,

$x^3 = A^3[\sin^3(2\pi f1t) + \sin^3(2\pi f2t) + 3\sin(2\pi f1t)\sin^2(2\pi f2t) + 3\sin(2\pi f2t)\sin^2(2\pi f1t)]$

$\sin^3(2\pi f1t) = 1/4[3\sin(2\pi f1t) - \sin(2\pi(3*f1)t)]$

$\sin^3(2\pi f2t) = 1/4[3\sin(2\pi f2t) - \sin(2\pi(3*f2)t)]$

$3\sin(2\pi f1t)\sin^2(2\pi f2t) = 3/4[\cos(2\pi f1t) - \cos(2\pi(f1+2f2)t) - \cos(2\pi(f2+2f1)t]$

$3\sin(2\pi f2t)\sin^2(2\pi f2t) = 3/4[\cos(2\pi f1t) - \cos(2\pi(f1-2f2)t) - \cos(2\pi(f2-2f1)t]$

Thus, *3f1, 3f2, 2f1+f2, 2f2+f1, 2f1-f2,* and *2f2-f1* are all now present in the nonlinear output, y.

Chapter 14 - Auditory Perception and Sound Source Determination

CD-ROM, Web Site, ASA Tapes: The CD-ROM and Web Site (*www.parmly.luc.edu/*) should be consulted.
<u>ASA Tapes:</u> Demonstration 39, Track 80.

Instructional Hints: Al Bregman in his book *Auditory Scene Analysis* (MIT Press, 1990) uses the analogy to a visual scene to describe sound source determination. For sound we perceive an auditory scene where each image represents a sound source. The auditory periphery does not produce this auditory scene. It is produced by the many neural circuits of the brain. The recognition that hearing might be defined as sound source determination was made during the middle of the 1800s, but was not a dominant theme in hearing until recently. Fascination with the incredible ability of the auditory system to determine a sound's frequency and the remarkable function of the auditory periphery dominated auditory science for most of the 20th century. Thus, not a great deal is known about how the auditory system processes the information from a sound source and from multiple sound sources. Chapter 14 in the Textbook is an attempt to describe some of the work in auditory perception that relates to sound source determination, rather than attempting to describe how it occurs.

An interesting discussion with students might occur if a piece of music containing several different instruments is played from a single loudspeaker. If the students are asked to name the instruments they will usually do a good job. An interesting set of answers occurs if you then ask what the sound source is for this piece of music. Most students will tend to give the same answers as before, that is, they name the instruments. But, in a very real sense the sound source is the loudspeaker. That is, there are no instruments. Thus, the output of the loudspeaker is like the sound field described in Chapters 1 and 14 in the Textbook. The single sound field coming from the loudspeaker arrives at the ears of the listeners. Additional discussion about how the sound field is processed by the inner ear and auditory nerve should help generate insights concerning the importance of the brainstem and auditory cortex for determining the instruments. Additional discussion about localization and determining the instruments often leads to further insights. That is, interaural differences might allow the students to know where in the room the loudspeaker is located, but not where any instrument was located in the original band or orchestra.

Speech is a very important complex sound for humans. The Textbook cannot cover speech production and perception in much depth. Any computer program or other product that produces artificial speech often makes a good vehicle for describing speech production. Another interesting discussion can center on the degree to which speech is a special (perhaps unique) waveform for humans as opposed to a highly over-learned complex waveform that is basically similar to any other complex sound. The work of Watson and colleagues on auditory patterns, briefly described in Chapter 14 in the Textbook, is one experimental attempt at investigating these issues.

Chapter 14-Suggested Problems for Students

1) You are at a party and you hear your friend talking, the music playing, and the door opening and closing as other guests come and go. What are the sources for the sounds that you are "hearing"? Does each sound arrive at your "ears" as a separate acoustic event? Explain.

2) For problem 1), what characteristics of the sound produced by each source might allow the auditory system to determine each sound source? Is it likely that cochlear processes are mainly responsible for determining the sound sources that you perceive at this party? Explain.

3) Figure 15.1 in the Textbook describes a simulation of the spectral-temporal code that might be generated in the cochlea and passed on to the central auditory nervous system by the auditory nerve. At the end of Chapter 9 in the Textbook, Figures 9.13-9.14 display similar types of cochlear representation for a single vowel sound. These figures and the discussion in the Textbook suggest a limitation that exists if the cochlear code for sounds is based only on firing rate. What is that limitation and how might it influence the ability of the auditory system to determine sound sources in a complex acoustic environment?

4) Two different sound sources can produce sounds with very similar spectra. The audible difference between the two sounds may be based on a change in the energy of a single spectral component of the sound. Yet, we can perceive a difference between these two sounds when they are loud and also when they are soft. Describe how the work on *profile analysis* helps explain how the auditory system might analyze these two sounds.

5) Explain what might happen in problem 4) to one's ability to discriminate a difference between the two sounds if only five or six spectral components were present in the spectra of the two sounds as compared to ten to twelve spectral components.

6) A music synthesizer produces two musical-like sounds, one with a spectrum consisting of 333, 666, 999, and 1332 Hz and the other consisting of 900, 1350, 1800, and 2250 Hz. If these two musical sounds were played together would one be likely to perceive one musical-like sound or two musical-like sounds? Explain.

7) Two sound sources are three feet apart. It is crucial that the sound of one of the sources is detected. If the sound sources were separated by a greater distance would it assist the detection of the sound from the crucial sound source? Explain. Your explanation should consider the *MLD* effect and the relative interaural differences of time and level that are likely to exist when the two sound sources are moved further apart.

8) Define *fusion* and *segregation*.

9) Why does listening to music through a single headphone suggest that spatially separating sounds cannot be the entire reason for sound source segregation?

10) As you listen to a TV program, a car with a loud muffler sound appears down the street. Describe how *fusion* and *segregation* aid in your ability to perceive both sound sources.

11) Recall that a melody is a series of musical notes played in succession. Use the idea of *auditory stream analysis* to describe why you might be able to hear two different melodies when they are played at the same time.

12) How does one's ability to discriminate a change in one part of a complex sound depend on the *uncertainty* of the listening task?

13) What is the difference between *informational masking* and the type of masking described in the masking chapter in the Textbook, Chapter 11?

14) In some situations the threshold of a signal tone masked by a noise masker is lower when the noise is on continuously and the tone is turned on and off than when the noise and tone are turned on and off together. What characteristic of sound source determination may help explain this difference in masked threshold? Explain your answer.

15) Compare and contrast the stimulus conditions that yield *CMR* and *MDI* and also describe the differences in the results.

16) Consider a masking experiment in which a complex masker consisted of two tones of different frequencies and the signal was a tone with the frequency of one of the maskers. Which condition might produce the lowest signal threshold and why?

   A) Both masker tones were modulated with the same pattern of amplitude modulation.

   B) Both masker tones were modulated but with different patterns of amplitude modulation.

   C) Only one of the masker tones was an amplitude-modulated tone.

   D) Neither of the masker tones was an amplitude-modulated tone.

17) Describe the basic process of producing speech.

18) What is the basic auditory unit of speech?

19) What are *formants* and how are they determined?

20) What is a basic acoustic difference between a vowel like /e/ as in the word "bead" and a consonant such as the letter "b?"

21) In a *speech spectrograph* describe what each of the three axises depict.

22) Why might continuous discourse be more difficult for computer speech recognition than the recognition of isolated words?

23) How does the two-vowel recognition procedure allow one to study sound source segregation?

ADVANCED PROBLEMS

1) How does *pulsation threshold* differ from *auditory stream analysis*?

2) Why isn't FM itself a useful cue for sound source determination?

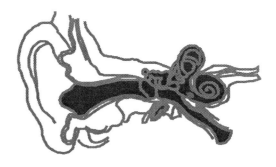

Answers for Problems for CHAPTER 14

1) No, each sound does not travel to the ear of a listener directly from the source. All sounds are combined into a single vibratory pattern that moves the tympanic membrane. In most acoustic environments, the sounds from the different sound sources will also encounter various obstacles as they travel and these obstacles will affect the sound (e.g., cause a reflection).

2) There are seven possible physical cues that have been suggested that might aid the auditory system in determining sound sources: *Spectral Separation, Spectral Profile, Harmonicity, Spatial Separation, Temporal Separation, Temporal Onsets and Offsets,* and *Temporal Modulations.* Cochlear mechanisms appear to code for the spectral-temporal properties of the entire complex sound field reaching the auditory system and not for sound sources per se.

3) Nerve fibers in the auditory nerve appear to have a saturation rate at moderate sound pressure levels indicating that firing rate cannot increase much beyond the saturation rate as the stimulus level is increased to higher levels. Thus, at a high stimulus level most fibers will be firing near or at their saturation rate. At high levels, then, the entire auditory nerve is likely to be stimulated near saturation, even if the stimulus only contains a limited range of frequencies. Thus, at high levels the spectral aspect of the code is likely to be lost.

4) *Profile analysis* suggests that the auditory system can compare the <u>relative</u> levels of different spectral components that make up a complex sound. The relative levels of the various components of a complex sound will not change if the overall level of the entire sound is changed. Thus, if one sound has one relationship among the relative levels of its spectral components that differs from the relationship of the relative levels of a different complex sound, then the auditory system could distinguish between the two sounds, even if the overall level of the sounds is varied.

5) According to Figure 14.4 in the Textbook, the ability to determine the *spectral profile* of a complex sound with five or six spectral components is poorer than for a stimulus with ten to twelve spectral components. Thus, one would predict that the ability to discriminate between two complex sounds with five or six components would be worse than for ten to twelve components.

6) The sound with the harmonics of 333 Hz would produce a single pitch of 333 Hz if it were presented alone. The other stimulus has a "missing fundamental" of 450 Hz, and would likely produce a single pitch of 450 Hz if it were presented alone. However, if the two complex harmonic stimuli were summed and presented without any other differences, it is likely that a single musical-like sound would be heard, since the auditory system does not usually analyze such complex sounds into two harmonic structures.

7) Yes, it would probably help if the two sound sources were moved further apart. In this case the interaural differences of time and level would be increased for one sound source relative to the other.

Work on the *MLD* suggests that if the interaural differences of time and level for one stimulus are different from those of another stimulus, then it is easier to detect one stimulus in the presence of the other stimulus.

8) *Fusion* is the ability of the auditory system to form one sound source from an array of acoustical information. *Segregation* is the ability to form separate sound sources (each fused).

9) When one listens to music through one headphone and if one can determine the different instruments or voices (the different sound sources) in the music, then it is unlikely that binaural cues like the interaural differences of time and level are necessary and sufficient for sound source determination. That is, since only one ear is being stimulated there are no interaural differences that would facilitate the spatial separation of the various instruments and voices. Other cues must be available to allow the auditory system to determine these sound sources.

10) *Fusion* means that the auditory system can combine all of the spectral-temporal information associated with one sound (say the music) so that this sound source is perceived. So *fusion* would allow one to perceive the music and the muffler sound if each was presented by itself. When they are presented together, *segregation* refers to the ability of the auditory system to separate the two fused sound images into two perceived sound sources.

11) The spectral and temporal structure of one melody may allow it to be fused into an *auditory stream* that is different from the perceived *auditory stream* associated with the other melody. *Stream segregation* would be assisted if the two melodies were played in different frequency regions, with different overall levels, with different timbres (e.g., with different instruments), or were played to different ears (e.g., allowing for spatial separation).

12) If the base stimulus for which one is trying to determine a change is itself changing from moment to moment (from trial to trial in an experimental context), then this *uncertainty* about the base stimulus makes it difficult to discern small changes to the stimulus. The less *uncertainty* there is about the base stimulus, the better one can discern small changes in the stimulus.

13) The masking discussed elsewhere in the Textbook is that presumably due to the direct interaction of the sounds at the auditory periphery (e.g., in the auditory nerve). Such interactions are predictable on the basis of the *energy* in the stimulus in different frequency regions (e.g., sounds close together in frequency are more likely to mask one another than if they were further apart in frequency). *Informational masking* refers to cases in which one might not predict much masking based on the energy distribution of the stimuli. The uncertainty about the spectral-temporal structure of the stimulus from moment to moment leads to more masking than predicted on the basis of the distribution of *energy* in the stimuli.

14) *Onset and offset differences in time* of presentation of one sound relative to that of another sound can aid in sound source segregation. Thus, if a signal is pulsed on or off at a different time than a masker, then one might predict less masking than if the signal and masker were pulsed on and off at the same time.

15) *CMR or comodulation masking release* refers to the increased ability to detect a signal in the presence of multiple maskers, when the maskers have coherent or comodulated amplitude envelopes (i.e., when the maskers are coherently amplitude modulated) as compared to cases in which the maskers' envelopes are not comodulated. *MDI or modulation detection interference* refers to the decrease in ability to detect a change in amplitude modulation of one sound in the presence of another sound when both are comodulated as compared to cases in which the two sounds are not comodulated. Thus, *CMR* indicates an improvement in performance based on comodulation, whereas *MDI* indicates a decrement in performance based on comodulation. Both cases suggest that sounds that are amplitude comodulated are processed more as a single sound source than when they are not comodulated. In *CMR*, the comodulation maskers are perceived as one sound source, making it easier to discern the signal as a separate sound source. In *MDI*, the comodulated stimuli are perceived as a single sound source, making it difficult to discern a difference in the modulation pattern of this single source.

16) Case A describes the *CMR* condition that tends to yield best detection. That is, both maskers are comodulated. Thus, this condition would be predicted to yield the lowest threshold.

(For the advanced student: When the signal tone that is not amplitude modulated is added to a masker tone of the same frequency that is amplitude modulated, the depth of modulation of the signal-plus-masker stimulus is reduced. Thus, the task in Case A might be described as one of detecting which stimulus has a lower depth of amplitude modulation. The signal-plus-masker stimulus will have a lower depth of modulation than the masker alone stimulus. Thus, viewed in this way the task is more like an *MDI* task than a *CMR* task. As such, Case A would not be predicted to produce the lowest threshold. The prediction one might make when both the *CMR and MDI* approaches are considered depends on the signal level that might be used. The interested student should consult Yost, Sheft, and Opie, J. Acoust. Soc. Am 86, 2138-2148, 1989, for a paper describing a similar set of experiments.)

17) Speech starts with the air produced by the diaphragm pushing on the *vocal cords* producing a pulsating sound that is further spectrally shaped by the *vocal tract*. The parts of the *vocal tract* such as the throat, mouth, libs, tongue, and nasal passages provide different resonators which filter the voiced sound of the *vocal cords*. The vocal cords produce the fundamental vibratory voice frequency, which determines the pitch of a voice. The *vocal tract* controls the dynamic changes in speech that results in the articulated *phonemes* of speech.

18) The *phoneme* is usually referred to as the basic unit of speech.

19) *Formants* are spectral peaks of energy in the spectrum of speech that are associated with particular vocal-tract resonators. *Formants* determine the different phonemes of speech.

20) The *vowel* /e/ is steady state in that the waveform does not change over time. An /e/ is perceived the same no matter how long it is sounded. A *consonant* such as "b" contains a *formant transition* from the first part of the sound to the last part of the sound. A *consonant* is a dynamic speech sound in that its acoustic characteristics change over time.

21) In a speech *spectrograph* the x-axis is usually time, the y-axis is amplitude or level, and the z-axis is frequency or spectral region.

22) In continuous discourse the computer needs to recognize the difference between boundaries between words as opposed to boundaries between phonemes or smaller segments of speech. Word boundaries signify a different aspect of the meaning of speech than boundaries between phonemes.

23) Being able to identify two vowel sounds in a mixture is like identifying two sound sources.

ADVANCED PROBLEMS

1) *Pulsation threshold* refers to perception of continuity of one repeating sound in the presence of another repeating sound. While the continuous sound may be perceived as a separate sound source than the other pulsating sound, it is not necessary for the estimate of pulsation threshold for there to be a perception of different sound sources. In *auditory stream analysis*, the two sounds are separated as if there were two sound sources. Also, in stream segregation neither pulsating sound appears as if it were continuous.

2) FM can also lead to differences in harmonicity. Thus, harmonicity and not FM per se may be the basis for sound source determination and segregation.

Chapter 15 - The Central Auditory Nervous System

CD-ROM, Web Site, ASA Tapes: The CD-ROM and Web Site (*www.parmly.luc.edu/*) should be consulted.

Instructional Hints: The study of the central auditory nervous system could be a course in itself. Thus, the coverage in *Fundamentals of Hearing: An Introduction* is minimal. One difficulty in presenting material on the CANS is the lack of a clear understanding of the function of each CANS nucleus. The approach taken in the Textbook is to first provide some information about how people have studied the CANS and then to provide the basic anatomy and physiology of some of the most studied CANS nuclei. When possible a functional description of the nucleus is provided as in the case of the MSO and LSO, which appear to be clearly involved with sound localization. Appendix F is highly recommended since many of these techniques are those used to study the CANS.

Students are often overwhelmed by the complexity of the CANS and the lack of clear functional descriptions make the complexity even more difficult to master. Perhaps this complexity is due to the enormous calculations that the CANS must perform. Take the use of interaural time and level as cues for horizontal sound localization as an example. These interaural differences must be computed from the neural information arriving at the MSO and LSO from the two cochlear nuclei. Then the outcome of the calculations must be arranged in some sort of neural circuit (perhaps in the inferior colliculus) that corresponds to horizontal space. This would appear to require a fairly big computer.

It is important for the student to appreciate that just determining how cells within the CANS are interconnected is a major task. Then characterizing the physiology of single units in the CANS is also not easy. But, these single units must operate in some sort of neural circuit which demands understanding how single units interact. There is very little knowledge about those interactions, mainly because there are not good techniques to study multiple neurons. This is one of the reasons that slice preparations are often used. Even though the slice is not in a functioning animal, the slice preparation does allow one to investigate cellular interactions.

As one ascends toward the cortex the role of anesthesia becomes more important. Anesthesia acts on the efferent system and often "quiets" the neural actions that might normally take place. Thus, one may find very little neural activity in a CANS region, not because the region is unresponsive to the auditory stimulus, but because the anesthesia used in the experiment has affected this neural region. Recent animal models, like the rabbit, which enable one to use chronic recording techniques in awake animals, offer a real advantage for studying certain aspects of neural function.

Chapter 15- Suggested Problems for Students

1) At the end of this chapter is a diagram that can be used to test students on their knowledge of the central auditory nervous system.

2) What are the major auditory nuclei of the ascending auditory pathway?

3) Define:
    A) *contralateral* B) *ipsilateral* C) *collaterals* D) *first-order fiber* E) *fibers of passage*
    F) *inter-neurons* G) *tonotopic organization* H) *bilateral*

4) What is the apparent primary physiological function of the descending auditory pathway?

5) What is meant when a neural unit is said to be "tuned" to a particular stimulus parameter?

6) What are the differences between *E-E* and *E-I* cells?

7) Name one excitatory and one inhibitory *neurotransmitter*.

8) In Chapter 15 in the Textbook, show the mathematics that yields the levels of excitation for each of the seven output neurons shown in Fig. 15.7.

9) Use these labels to identify each neuronal type shown below. *primary-like, phasor-on, phasor-off, on-off, inhibitory, tonic, chopper*

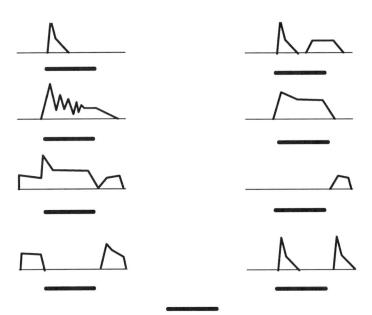

Stimulus on-off

10) What is the *CF* of the fiber whose *PST* is shown below? Is this fiber likely to be from the *auditory nerve* or the *cochlear nucleus*? Why?

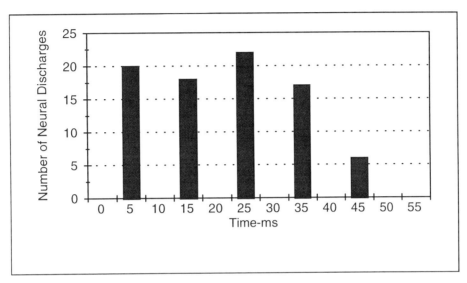

11) A physiologist has data from two different neurons; she knows that one neuron was from the *cochlear nucleus* and the other from the *inferior colliculus*. The latency from stimulus onset to the first neural activity from neuron A is 8 ms, while the latency for neuron B is 13 ms. Which neuron is likely to be from the *inferior colliculus*? Why?

12) What is an *auditory evoked potential*?

13) The data on the next page are from five presentations of the same stimulus. Each data point is the magnitude (in millivolts) of evoked neural activity recorded from a pair of scalp electrodes. The voltage is shown as a function of time in ms. What is the evoked potential for this condition?

Table(next page). The voltages (millivolts) of the evoked activity recorded from scalp electrodes are shown for ten points in time (in ms). The recorded voltages are shown for five stimulus presentations.

Time	1st Presentation	2nd Presentation	3rd Presentation	4th Presentation	5th Presentation
10 ms	0	2	-1	0	1
60 ms	3	8	3	5	4
110 ms	10	9	4	6	9
160 ms	5	3	-1	5	4
210 ms	2	-1	3	-2	2
260 ms	-1	-4	-3	-2	-1
310 ms	5	3	-1	-2	-2
360 ms	3	6	-7	8	-7
410 ms	2	3	-4	-3	3
460 ms	-4	-2	4	2	1

14) The latency of Wave V of the *BSER* was measured for four different intensities of a click stimulus. They were 8.2 ms, 6.1 ms, 7.3 ms, and 7 ms. The four intensities were 30, 40, 50, and 60 dB SPL. Plot the relationship between Wave V latency (in ms) and stimulus level (in dB SPL) that you would expect to find for such an experiment. The latencies and levels shown above are not in any order. You are to use your knowledge of the *BSER* to plot the data.

15) What are the main divisions of the *cochlear nucleus*?

16) Name four of the cell types found in the *cochlear nucleus*?

17) The various cell types in the *cochlear nucleus* have different appearances (morphologies). Do they also have different physiological properties? If so, give an example of how a physiological property differs between two different cell types. That is, choose a physiological property and two different cell types and describe how the physiological property differs between the two cell types.

18) Describe in general terms the *tonotopic organization* of the *AVCN*.

19) What are the four major nuclei of the *superior olivary complex*?

20) What appears to be the main function of the *MSO* and of the *LSO*? Describe some of the physiological evidence that supports your description of the function of the *MSO* and *LSO*.

21) What are the three major areas of the *inferior colliculus*?

22) Does the *IC* have more *E-E* or *E-I* cell types?

23) Suppose that some cells in the *IC* fired best to a particular delay between a stimulus delivered to the left and right ears (i.e., the cells demonstrated *characteristic delays*). What aspect of auditory perception might these cells be responsible for? Explain your answer.

24) Describe the general tonotopic organization of the *auditory cortex*.

25) Why is it difficult to study the *auditory cortex* in primates, but easier in cats?

26) An experimenter used tonal stimuli to study single neurons in the auditory cortex. He found that almost none of the neurons responded to the tones no matter what frequencies or overall levels he tried. He concluded that his equipment must be broken. Is there any other reason why the cortical neurons might not have responded to the tones?

27) What is an *ablation study* and how can it provide information about what type of information the *cortex* or part of the cortex processes?

Answers for Problems for CHAPTER 15

2) In ascending order: cochlear nucleus, olivary complex, lateral lemniscus, inferior colliculus, medial geniculate, auditory cortex.

3)   A) *contralateral*: Side opposite
      B) *ipsilateral*: On the same side
      C) *collaterals*: Fibers that branch out from the main nerve track
      D) *first-order fiber*: Fibers after the first synapse from the periphery. In the auditory system those fibers in the cochlear nucleus.
      E) *fibers of passage*: Fibers that pass through a nucleus without synapsing with cells in the nucleus.
      F) *inter-neurons*: Neurons that connect one fiber to another within the same nucleus.
      G) *tonotopic organization*: The neural organization of fibers based on the frequency to which the fibers is tuned.
      H) *bilateral*: Inputs from both sides of the brain (or ear).

4) The descending pathways modify the neural information provided by the ascending pathways. They do so by inhibitory or excitatory action at the synapses and on the axons of the ascending fibers.

5) Tuning means that the fiber responds with the highest firing rate to a particular value of a stimulating variable. For instance, if the fiber responds with the highest firing rate to a tone of a particular frequency then the fiber is tuned to that frequency, if it fires with the highest firing rate to a modulated tone with a particular modulation rate, then it is tuned to the modulation rate, etc. The implication is that the fiber is carrying information about that stimulus value for use by other parts of the auditory system.

6) *E-E* cells are cells that receive two inputs and the cell's output is determined by the two inputs both being excitatory, that is, the cell produces a discharge as if it were adding the two inputs. For *E-I* cells there are also two inputs and one is excitatory and the other inhibitory, that is, the cell produces a discharge as if it were subtracting the two inputs.

7) Inhibitory neurotransmitters include: *amino acids* such as *gamma-aminobutyric acid (GABA)* and *glycine*. Excitatory neurotransmitters include: *acetylcholine*.

8) Starting on the left:
Input of 5x1 - inhibition from both sides of (.2x5 +.2x5) = output of 3
Input of 5x1 - inhibition from both sides of (.2x5 +.2x10) = output of 2
Input of 10x1 - inhibition from both sides of (.2x10 +.2x5) = output of 7
Input of 10x1 - inhibition from both sides of (.2x10 +.2x10) = output of 6

Input of 10x1 - inhibition from both sides of (.2x5 +.2x10) = output of 7
Input of 5x1 - inhibition from both sides of (.2x10 +.2x5) = output of 2
Input of 5x1 - inhibition from both sides of (.2x5 +.2x5) = output of 3

9)

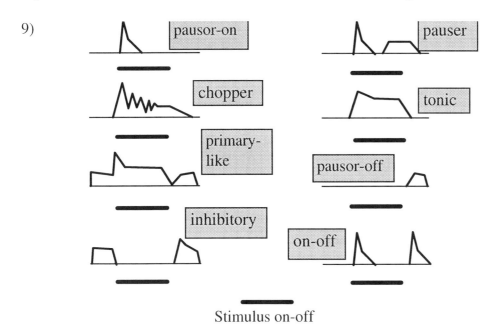

Stimulus on-off

10) The center frequency (*CF*) of the fiber is likely to be 100 Hz since the fiber tends to fire every 10 ms (1/10ms =100 Hz), and the fiber is likely to be an auditory nerve fiber rather than a cochlear nucleus fibers since the *PST* shows the modulated *PST* pattern at a rate of 1/*CF*.

11) Since the *inferior colliculus* is at least one synapse higher in the auditory system than the *cochlear nucleus*, it will take longer for a neural response to be initiated; thus, neuron B is from the *inferior colliculus* and neuron A from the *cochlear nucleus*.

12) An *auditory evoked potential* is the average *electroencephalogram (EEG)* recording generated by repeated stimulation by the same auditory stimulus. The *auditory evoked potential* presumably represents cortical activity evoked by the particular stimulus.

13)

Time	1st	2nd	3rd	4th	5th	*Total*	*Average*
10 ms	0	2	-1	0	1	2	*0.4*
60 ms	3	8	3	5	4	23	*4.6*
110 ms	10	9	4	6	9	38	*7.6*
160 ms	5	3	-1	5	4	16	*5.2*
210 ms	2	-1	3	-2	2	4	*0.8*
260 ms	-1	-4	-3	-2	-1	-11	*–2.2*
310 ms	5	3	-1	-2	2	7	*-1.4*
360 ms	3	6	-7	8	-7	3	*0.6*
410 ms	2	3	-4	-3	3	1	*0.2*
460 ms	-4	-2	4	2	1	1	*0.2*

The *Average Value*s would represent the *evoked potential,* suggesting that a peak in the evoked potential occurred in the time period around 110 ms.

14) Since the latency of the *BSER* depends directly on stimulus intensity, the data need to be arranged in order of stimulus intensity. When that is done, the following graph would reflect the *BSER* waveform.

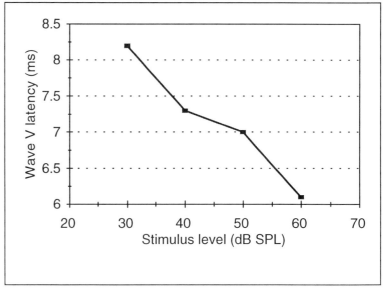

15) *Dorsal Cochlear Nucleus (DCN), Anteroventral Cochlear Nucleus (AVCN),* and *Posteroventral Cochlear Nucleus (PVCN).*

16) The cell types in the *cochlear nucleus* are: *primary-like cells, spherical bushy cells, globular bushy cells, stellite cells, multipolar cells, octopus cells, globular cells,* and *fusiform cells.*

17) Refer to Figure 15.14 (see also Figure 15.4) in the Textbook. *Spherical bushy cells* in the *AVCN* have only excitatory tuning curves (far right-hand side of Fig. 15.14), while *fusiform cells* in the *DCN* may have only small areas of excitation and inhibition (far right-hand side of Fig. 15.14).

18) The *AVCN* is *tonotopically* organized such that high frequencies are coded toward the *DCN* end of the *cochlear nucleus* and the *CF* of fibers decrease in frequency as the neurons appear more toward the region where the *auditory nerve* enters the *cochlear nucleus.*

19) The *superior olivary complex* consists of the *lateral superior olive,* the *medial superior olive,* the *trapezoid body,* and the *preolivary nuclei.*

20) The *MSO* appears to process interaural time differences, while the *LSO* processes interaural level differences. The *MSO* has *E-E cells,* low-frequency CFs, and units which exhibit *characteristic delays,* all of which are consistent with coding for interaural time differences. The *LSO* has *E-I* cells, high-frequency CFs, and is differentially sensitive to interaural level differences, all of which are consistent with coding for interaural level differences.

21) The three regions of the *IC* are: *central nucleus, dorsal cortex,* and *paracentral nucleus.*

22) More cells seem to be of the *E-I* type than of the *E-E* type in the *IC.*

23) *Characteristic delay* for an interaural time difference would suggest that the neural unit is aiding in sound localization.

24) Cells with similar CFs tend to lie in *cortical* columns that are perpendicular to the *cortical* surface.

25) The *auditory cortex* is located deeper within the *cortex* in cats than it is in primates, making it easier to reach in cats.

26) If anesthetics were used they may have shut off efferent inputs and thus make it difficult to find *cortical* units that would respond to sounds. Also, many *cortical* units discharge to complex sounds, but not to simple sinusoidal sounds.

27) An *ablation* means that some part of the nervous system is removed (or sometimes made to be neurally inactive), so a *cortical ablation* means that some part of the *cortex* was removed. By studying how an animal's behavior is modified as a result of the *ablation,* one might be able to determine the functional significance of the part of the *cortex* that was *ablated.*

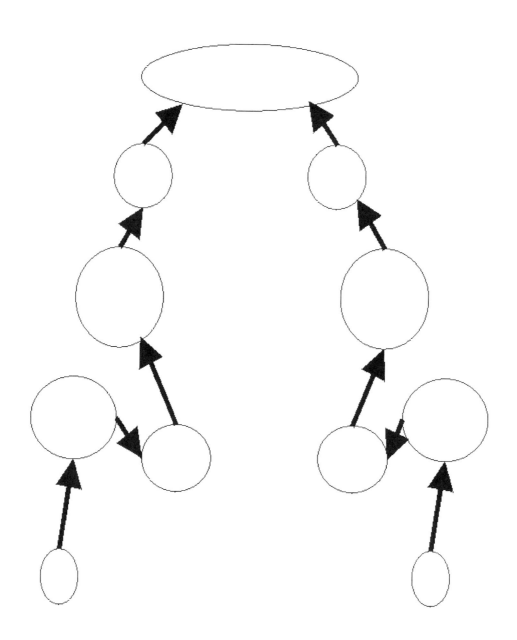

Chapter 16 - The Abnormal Auditory System

CD-ROM, Web Site, ASA Tapes: The CD-ROM and Web Site (*www.parmly.luc.edu/*) should be consulted.

Instructional Hints: As mentioned in the Textbook, Chapter 16 is not intended to be a thorough review of the abnormal auditory system. Students should appreciate that studying normal and abnormal auditory systems and processing is a two-way street. Each helps one understand the other. A great deal is known about noise exposure and this knowledge has helped in understanding hearing loss and in how the cochlea functions. Since little is known about the exact function of neural centers above the auditory periphery, it is difficult to identify what hearing problems might develop if a particular CANS nucleus was damaged. If one could find that a particular hearing problem was correlated with damage to a particular nucleus, then this would be crucial data indicating the possible function of that nucleus.

Noise pollution is a major environmental topic. Many standards exist concerning permissible noise levels in the workplace and for places like airports. These standards are based both on TTS data and on data concerning the levels and types of noise that are annoying and disrupt other functions like sleep and speech communication. There is no doubt that exposure to loud sounds will increase the rate at which one losses hearing sensitivity with age. Thus, excessive "Walkman" use is a health hazard.

Ototoxic drugs like the aminoglycosides have been valuable in studying haircell function. Since with proper delivery and dosage these drugs can selectively destroy haircells, one can study the consequences of haircell damage. The same thing can be done with sound exposure, but ototoxic drugs are often easier to administer and they can provide more "pinpoint" destruction than that achieved as a result of noise exposure.

The understanding of the genetic make up of the auditory system is likely to be the next revolution in understanding hearing. Not only will inheritable diseases and conditions be better understood and perhaps cured, but things like neural repair (e.g., haircell regeneration) might be possible. However, genetics by itself is not likely to solve problems like understanding the function of CANS nuclei. It is more and more evident that understanding big questions like that will require a multidisciplinary and interdisciplinary approach.

Neural plasticity is a major topic in neuroscience and is in some sense the basis of learning and memory. Far less has been done in hearing than has been done in other areas like vision. Part of the reason deals with the fact that so little is known about the function of the various CANS brain centers. Most has been done with sound localization, since most is known about the neural centers that play a role in sound localization.

Chapter 16-Suggested Problems for Students

1) What are the ways in which the normal auditory system can become abnormal?

2) Differentiate between *PTS* and *TTS*. What are *ATS* and *CTS*?

3) What is probably the most fragile part of the *inner ear* than can fail and lead to *NIHL*?

4) A person has a hearing loss in the region of 4,000 Hz and the audiologist is almost certain that it was due to exposure to loud sounds. What is your best guess as to the frequencies of the sounds that lead to the hearing loss and why?

5) If you could examine the *haircells* of the patient described in problem 4, under what conditions might you expect to find *haircell* damage, what kind of damage might you find for each condition, and where along the *basilar membrane* might the *haircell* damage occur?

6) A gunshot is a broad-spectrum sound with sound energy spread somewhat evenly across a wide range of frequencies. If someone is exposed to high-levels of gunshot sounds, in what frequency region might one expect to find a hearing loss as measured by *TTS*?

7) According to the *5-dB rule*, how many decibels of *TTS* might I have after 10 hours of exposure to a loud sound, if after 5 hours I had 14 decibels of *TTS*?

8) About how long does it take to reach 100% of the TTS that one might ever acquire?

9) A person is exposed to a high-level, pure tone with a frequency of 2,000 Hz. In what frequency range might you expect to find a hearing loss?

10) People who work in a certain factory are exposed to high-level sounds in the region of 1,000 to 2,000 Hz. After several of these factory workers had died, autopsies were performed and *cochleograms* were obtained. What might one expect to find in these *cochleograms?*

11) What drugs are *ototoxic* to *haircells*?

12) What is *tinnitus* and is there a cure for it?

13) Why would people with arthritis who take large doses of aspirin have to see an otologist or audiologist?

14) What is *presbycusis*?

15) What is *otitis media* and why is it potentially dangerous?

16) Briefly describe *otosclerosis* and *Menieres disease*.

17) Name one disease condition that appears to be inherited?

18) Describe how *inner* and *outer haircell* loss differentially affects auditory sensitivity and frequency resolution.

19) A person is tested and it is found that she is not as sensitive to sound as a person with normal hearing, but her ability to differentiate tones of different frequencies is near normal. What type of *haircell* loss might she have? Eːplain.

20) Mammalian *haircells* do not regenerate. Is this true for all animals? Please explain your answer. If not all animals permanently lose *haircells*, why is this important for future treatments of hearing loss?

21) What is neural *plasticity*?

22) One group of animals is reared in a situation in which they never received high-frequency sounds. A physiologist compares the *tonotopic* organization of auditory cortex of these animals to the auditory cortex of another group of animals that were reared with equal exposure to all frequencies. If the auditory cortex demonstrated *plasticity* to frequency processing, what might the physiologist find when comparing the cortical *tonotopic* organization of the two groups of animals?

Answers for Problems for CHAPTER 16

1) Noise *exposure, age, drugs, disease* and *infections, accidents*, and *heredity* can lead to an abnormal auditory system.

2) *PTS* stands for permanent threshold shift, which is a hearing loss that never recovers. *TTS* is a temporary hearing loss, which is a hearing loss that does recover over time. *ATS* is the asymptotic or maximum temporary threshold shift that can result from *TTS*, while *CTS* is compound threshold shift which results from a combination of *TTS* and *PTS*.

3) *Haircells* and their *stereocillia* are the most fragile part of the *cochlea*.

4) Sounds in the region of 4,000 Hz or higher probably lead to a 4,000-Hz hearing loss, since *TTS* usually occurs near the frequency of the exposure sound are at higher frequencies.

5) If the sound was intense, the *haircells* may be completely missing and the missing *haircells* would be in a region of the cochlea that was associated with coding the frequency of the exposing sound. At lower levels of exposure the *haircells* may be present, but their *stereocillia* may be damaged in one way or another.

6) Figure 16.4 in the Textbook suggests that exposure to a broadband sound produces the most *TTS* in the frequency region between approximately 3 and 6 kHz.

7) The 5-dB rule suggests that for each doubling of exposure time, the amount of *TTS* increases by 5 dB. Thus, after 10 hours there would be 19 (14 + 5) decibels of *TTS*.

8) According to Figure 16.5 in the Textbook, it would take about 15 hours of exposure to reach 100% *ATS*.

9) High-level exposure to pure tones, produce the *half-octave shift*, which means that the hearing loss would be a half to a whole octave higher than 2,000 Hz or between 3,000 and 4,000 Hz.

10) The *cochleogram* would reveal *haircell* loss in a region of the *cochlea* that was associated with the coding of 1,000 to 2,000 Hz. This is near the middle toward the apical end of the *cochlea*, so one would expect to find significant *haircell* loss in the middle of the *cochlea* (15 to 20 mm from the base).

11) *Aminoglycosides* such as *kanamycin, neomycin*, and *streptomycin* are *ototoxic*.

12) *Tinnitus* is ringing in the ears or sounds that one hears when there is no apparent sound source. It is an abnormal condition for which there is no universal cure.

13) Aspirin contains *salicylate* and large doses of *salicylate* can lead to *tinnitus* and sometimes hearing loss.

14) *Presbycusis* is the loss of hearing due to aging.

15) *Otitis media* is infection of the *middle ear*. If left untreated and the infection gets into the *inner ear* it might lead to *meningitis,* which is a potentially deadly condition.

16) *Otosclerosis* is related to calcification of the *ossicular chain. Menieres disease* is a condition that affects the *inner ear* leading to balance and hearing difficulties.

17) *Usher's* and *Waardenberg Syndromes* are two conditions that appear to be inherited.

18) *Outer haircell* loss increases the sensitivity of the *tuning curve* causing a loss in sensitivity. The *tuning curve* also broadens and its *CF* moves to lower frequencies, resulting in a loss of frequency resolution. *Inner haircell* loss only causes a shift in the sensitivity of the *tuning curve*, without significant changes in its shape, probably resulting in a loss of sensitivity, but not a loss of frequency resolution. If both *inner* and *outer haircells* are lost then there is major shift in the sensitivity of the *tuning curve* and significant broadening, resulting in severe loss in both sensitivity and frequency resolution.

19) From the answer to problem 18, she probably suffered *inner haircell* loss.

20) Fish and birds' *haircells* tend to regenerate, but mammalian *haircells* do not. If a way can be found for mammalian *haircells* to regenerate then this would probably lead to a major "cure" for hearing loss given the crucial role *haircells* play in hearing.

21) *Neural plasticity* means changes in the anatomy or physiology due to a change in the stimulus conditions that an animal receives.

22) If *neural plasticity* occurs, then the cortical *tonotopic* organization should differ between the two groups. In most cases the *tonotopic* organization of the group that did not receive high-frequency sounds would have far fewer cells tuned to high frequencies than the group raised with exposure to all frequencies.